PREGNANT
ON **PROZAC**

PREGNANT ON PROZAC

The Essential Guide to
Making the Best Decision
for You and Your Baby

Shoshana S. Bennett, Ph.D.

Guilford, Connecticut
An imprint of The Globe Pequot Press

To buy books in quantity for corporate use
or incentives, call **(800) 962–0973**
or e-mail **premiums@GlobePequot.com.**

life

GPP Life gives women answers they can trust.

Copyright © 2009 by Shoshana S. Bennett

GPP Life is an imprint of The Globe Pequot Press.

Medical editor: Dr. Marlene P. Freeman
Text design by Sheryl P. Kober

Library of Congress Cataloging-in-Publication Data is available on file.

ISBN 978-0-7627-4940-9

Printed in the United States of America

10 9 8 7 6 5 4 3 2 1

CONTENTS

Contents

ACKNOWLEDGMENTS

I am especially grateful to:

Dr. Phyllis Cedars, psychiatrist, friend and colleague who, despite her packed schedule, always made time to give her honest and expert feedback.

Susan Stone, L.C.S.W., friend, perinatal expert, and trusted sounding board. No matter what the storms on the East Coast were doing to her computer and phone, she always came through.

Dr. Marlene P. Freeman, medical editor and internationally renowned researcher, who generously shared her expertise and opinions regarding the information presented.

Heather Carreiro, acquisitions editor, for her wisdom in understanding the timeliness of this book and for her trust in me to say what needed to be said.

Justine Rathbun, copy editor, for her detailed work and keen eye, and Himeka Curiel, project manager, for her suggestions and assistance.

Bob Sembiante, publicist, for ensuring that *Pregnant on Prozac* reaches all those who need it.

To mothers and their loved ones—those born and those not yet born. And to health professionals who care enough to find the best mental health treatments for their pregnant patients.

FOREWORD

I am honored that Dr. Shoshana Bennett has given me the opportunity to be a part of this valuable new resource for women. It is so important that women have information about pregnancy and mental wellness, yet there are too few reliable and accurate sources of information out there about this issue.

Since meeting Dr. Bennett in 2003, I continue to be impressed by her passion and commitment to an area that is still misunderstood and underestimated: postpartum depression. As the founder of the international organization, Postpartum Assistance for Mothers, Dr. Bennett has dedicated her time to educating the public about this important issue, revealing the many barriers that a woman faces when dealing with depression at a time when there is so much expectation for her to be happy.

Persuaded by Dr. Bennett's work, the Iris Alliance Fund—a mental health foundation I founded in 2001—conducted an opinion poll of 1,000 parents to learn more about attitudes and experiences with postpartum depression. The poll confirmed how common the problem was: More than half of those surveyed had either experienced postpartum depression themselves or knew someone who had. It also showed the need for more education to alleviate the needless suffering of women and their families; only 34 percent believed the disease was a major problem and more than a third would do nothing and wait for symptoms to pass if they thought they or their partner might have postpartum depression.

Dr. Bennett is determined to bring down the number of women who experience postpartum depression, as well as the number of those who try to ignore the disease rather than treat it. This book is a great step forward in that direction by filling a void in information for women who are pregnant or considering pregnancy when they have already been diagnosed with depression. For these women, there is a lot of confusion, guilt, and anxiety about how to continue treating their disease while pregnant, as well as about whether they will have to experience the same traumatic postpartum depression that they had with previous births.

Pregnant on Prozac serves to alleviate these worries, by educating prospective mothers about their treatment options, reassuring and empowering women to know that they can treat their disease and have a healthy pregnancy. The book speaks without judgment, providing an objective resource that encourages women and their partners to make informed decisions. Readers will find the real-life stories to be helpful and relevant, as relating personal experience does so much to bring home the message that taking care of a woman's mental health when she is considering pregnancy or is pregnant, should be just as important as taking care of her physical health.

The book's focus on the woman and her well-being means a lot to me. My older sister, Bo Yoon, died by suicide on

January 1, 1980, at the age of 17. While she was not pregnant or going through postpartum depression, she was experiencing many of the same pressures and sense of hopelessness that many women do all over the world. Growing up in Korea, it was not acceptable in our culture to talk about personal problems and to do so would bring shame upon the entire family. This stigma was so strong that just as my sister had no one to talk to about what she was going through, there was also no place in the family to talk about her death. In fact, it took me nearly twenty years to actually talk about what happened, especially in public.

That's why this book is so important. We need to end the stigma around mental health issues and bring these experiences out into the open. We need to understand that mothers and women who are pregnant can still have serious depression. And we—meaning partners, healthcare professionals, family members, and policymakers—have to ensure that their needs are taken care of. I would like to thank Dr. Bennett for continuing to end the stigma, and for advocating for women and their mental health with such heartfelt dedication.

—Assemblymember Mary Hayashi (D-18)
California State Legislature

INTRODUCTION

Until just a few years ago, women were told that pregnancy hormones would protect them from both physical and mental illness. Not only was this incorrect, but it caused untold suffering that lasted for generations. It's heartening that doctors and other health care professionals are now being taught otherwise, and needed treatment is available. Pregnant women and their families—including family members not yet born—no longer need to suffer with depression and other psychiatric disorders.

Mothers and mothers-to-be want to do the right thing for their babies and for themselves. By reading *Pregnant on Prozac*, you will soon see that you don't need to compromise your own well-being in order to take care of your baby. There is now solid information on a number of options that can be used to treat depression in pregnancy. Some of these can be used as stand-alone treatments, and others are used in combination to help ensure your health and that of your growing baby.

I'm a survivor of two life-threatening bouts of postpartum depression, neither of which was diagnosed. My well-meaning doctors and family had no idea how to help me. I was surrounded by ignorance and, unfortunately, a great deal of judgment. Intense fear and hopelessness consumed me on a daily basis, and the suffering continued off and on for years. Having experienced the power of these brain chemistry changes, I understand on a deep level how terrifying this can be when you don't know what's happening or what you can do to make it better. Years later, when I finally realized what this illness was, I started reading everything I could get my hands on from all over the world. Many other countries were light years ahead of the United States in the areas of diagnosis and treatment of depression and anxiety occurring postpartum. I also discovered that other countries were already aware that depression, anxiety, and other psychiatric disorders could also occur before the baby was born—in other words, during pregnancy. I promised myself that I would help other women and their families so that they didn't need to suffer the way my husband, children, and I had.

Since I first discovered that this devastating suffering was treatable (and often completely preventable), it's been my mission and my passion to educate medical and mental health professionals and the public about psychiatric disorders that occur during pregnancy and postpartum. Avoiding the disorders in the first place—prevention—whenever possible, is the name of the game.

Who Will Benefit from This Book

There is a huge need for a complete, balanced, and comprehensive guide for treatment options in pregnancy. The conflicting and often contradictory results of various studies can render any intelligent person cross-eyed with confusion. My intention is to provide a user-friendly reference book for the 15 to 21 percent of pregnant women already suffering, pregnant women who know they're high risk, and women who are thinking of getting pregnant. Even if you're not high risk, no one is immune to these disorders, and the better your wellness plan, the greater the chance for feeling healthy.

There are many options—both medical and nonmedical—to choose from when putting together a plan. The aim is to prevent you from having to surf around the Internet getting bombarded with so-called research, not knowing what to believe and what to ignore. *Pregnant on Prozac* has all the necessary up-to-date information that will help you make decisions about treatment—whether it's necessary now or it becomes necessary in the future.

Pregnant on Prozac outlines the trusted medical, alternative, and complementary therapies the field has to date. Although the literature on medications seems to change by the minute, this book will educate you to know where to look for the "real" scoop.

This concise book thoroughly discusses what your options are so that you and your practitioners can decide what will be most helpful and appropriate for *you*. There is no "one size fits all." What's right for you may not be right for the next person.

Stories and Quotes

Throughout the book, you'll find stories about my clients' personal experiences. These stories illustrate common worries, experiences, and situations with which you'll be able to identify. When I describe my clients' stories, you can be assured that they are quite real and true. Unlike most other authors, I do not believe in composite sketches—when bits and pieces of various people's stories are combined to look like one. That never feels authentic to me. In *Pregnant on Prozac*, you will hear one real woman's story at a time.

Finally, when there are quotes around a client's words, those are their actual words taken directly out of my notes during therapy sessions with them. The stories from the women who generously contributed to this book are truly their stories. Their names are changed for privacy's sake, but their words are their own.

A Few Words about Terminology

Please note that when I use the word *husband*, you can substitute "partner" for it (and vice-versa).

When I use the term *clinical expertise* or *clinical experience*, this means actual experience treating patients (or clients, as the case may be). For the purposes of this book, clinical expertise means the doctor or therapist has a strong professional background working with women in these particular situations. There are many excellent psychiatrists and other doctors who have taken courses and read about the topic of mood disorders in pregnancy (what I'll refer to as "book learning"), but this does not make them the kinds of experts that would be best for your situation. The most helpful professionals you can find for yourself are those who have had many years of experience actually treating women going through these illnesses. Ideally, your doctor would base treatment decisions on excellent research that leaves little doubt for questions about safety and mood outcomes.

Unfortunately, there has not been enough research on how best to treat pregnant women who suffer from mental health problems. Therefore, many of the most experienced of these doctors will know the research done in the area and its limitations, and feel comfortable prescribing psychiatric medications in creative ways for their patients, those not found in the medical texts yet. And, as with seasoned professionals in other fields, they will draw upon their experience and the research done in this area to help their patients make the most informed choices about treatment. That only comes with real life experience. In chapter 3 there is a list of four key questions to ask a prospective medical doctor, psychotherapist, or other practitioner to verify whether the professional has the appropriate background to help you.

Chapter 1

MAKING THE BIG DECISIONS

So you want to get pregnant—or maybe you already are—and you've got some very important decisions to make. You may have suffered from a mood disorder in the past; be currently dealing with depression, another mood disorder, or anxiety; or know you are high risk during pregnancy or postpartum. The kinds of decisions you're facing, such as whether to have a baby if you suffer from a mood disorder, whether to switch or stop medication in pregnancy, or whether to use alternative treatments in pregnancy, aren't like choosing which pair of shoes to wear in the morning. The process of making these types of decisions can feel overwhelming, and these decisions are complicated. After all, both your health and the health of your unborn child are involved, and you want to do the right thing. That takes thought, research, soul-searching, and finding the right professionals to trust. You deserve to congratulate yourself for picking up this book. Only a good mother-to-be would care enough about her health and the health of her child(ren) to use this resource and make sure she has at her fingertips the best information available.

What's a Mood Disorder?

Most people go through sad or elated moods from time to time, and that's normal. People with mood disorders (also called affective disorders), on the other hand, suffer from severe or prolonged mood states that get in the way of their daily functioning. Having a "down" or "blue" day once in a while, for instance, is not depression. In this society, it's common to hear things like, "My boyfriend and I had an argument. I'm so depressed!" The word depression *is thrown around to the point where many people think it just means a temporary funk. It doesn't. Depression, one of the most common mood disorders, is a serious illness, not simply a bit of temporary upset. Mood disorders involve a disturbance of mood (or a combination of irrationally happy [mania] and despondently sad [depression] moods, as in the case of bipolar disorder) that is not caused by any other physical or mental disorder. Among the general mood disorders classified in the fourth edition (1994) of the* Diagnostic and Statistical Manual of Mental Disorders *(DSM-IV) are major depressive disorder (serious depression), bipolar disorder (which used to be called manic depression), and dysthymia (a less severe but more chronic form of depression). You can see a list of the most common symptoms of bipolar disorder and depression in chapter 9.*

This chapter will hopefully make the beginning of this process easier for you. First I'll describe some of the specific situations that probably led you to pick up this book. Next, I'll discuss some of the major questions you're probably asking yourself and others around you. And finally, I'll give you some suggestions on how to go about actually making the right decisions for you, the pieces that are involved, and what your professional team will need to know in order to help guide you.

Various Scenarios

Ideally, each woman who is on a psychiatric medication or has needed one in the past will consult with her psychiatrist *before* becoming pregnant, so that a plan of action regarding whether and when to use a medication during pregnancy can be discussed. But often in the real world, even when birth control is used, a woman may suddenly find herself pregnant.

Approximately half of all pregnancies in the United States are not planned or not timed as the couple intended, leaving a lot of women facing sudden dilemmas about medications and treatment. If you find yourself unexpectedly pregnant and you are taking medication or struggling with depression, you are not alone. Your situation is very common.

You'll probably recognize yourself in one of the following situations. Even though one in particular might pertain specifically to you, I suggest you read them all. There will undoubtedly be tidbits of information in the other scenarios that you'll find helpful. The questions I've included in each scenario are some of the most common that I've heard over the last twenty years of working with pregnant women.

SCENARIO 1: I'M ON AN ANTIDEPRESSANT (OR OTHER PSYCHIATRIC MEDICATION) AND I'M PREGNANT.

"Has the medication already hurt the baby?" Some women are so worried about their medication possibly harming the fetus that they consider abortion. Please know that there is no need for alarm. And whatever you do, don't just stop your medication cold turkey! That can be dangerous for you and can cause serious relapse. There isn't one psychiatrist or researcher in the know who would say that the risk to the fetus is so great that you should terminate the pregnancy. Do your best to concentrate on dealing with the news about the pregnancy and put the medication question on a shelf until you've spoken with a knowledgeable professional. If you haven't already done so, contact the doctor who's prescribing your medication (preferably a psychiatrist) and arrange a consultation to discuss whether to stay on the medication or slowly wean off.

> Whatever you do, don't just stop your medication cold turkey!

"Emotionally I don't think I can handle the rest of this pregnancy. And even if I can get through the pregnancy, if I feel this bad now, how could I ever handle an infant in addition?" You may also have other children at home, making you doubt your ability to cope even further. If you feel terrible right now, it's understandable that you're thinking about doing whatever might stop the pain. That's a very natural reaction, so whether or not you were trying to get pregnant, please don't guilt-trip yourself if you're having thoughts about ending the pregnancy. It's also nothing personal against the baby. You're a woman in pain who simply wants the pain to stop.

Thoughts of terminating the pregnancy may go through

your head regardless of how much you had wanted the baby, which can be especially confusing when you've been trying to get pregnant for a while. Others may say, "But isn't this what you wanted? You should be happy!" And you long to be. They obviously don't understand what you're going through, which can be lonely. You need someone to talk to who is compassionate and won't punish you with their judgment or look at you quizzically for simply having the thought.

Then there is the issue of whether or not to actually terminate the pregnancy. A mother who would otherwise be thrilled about her pregnancy if she were not depressed may consider termination, and it is important that decisions about the pregnancy and motherhood are not driven by depression. Additionally, the relief that you are seeking and dreaming about probably won't happen the way you're envisioning if you actually abort. On top of that, you can be left with a postpartum depression or anxiety due to the biochemical reaction of the pregnancy ending.

Instead, what you desperately need and deserve at this point, as you're contemplating whether or not to continue the pregnancy, is both reassurance and someone knowledgeable who will back up that reassurance with a solid plan to help you. You need to know that you'll feel better with treatment for the rest of the pregnancy and also postpartum, and that you will feel like yourself again and be able to cope. Right now, you may not believe it's possible to feel well again, since depression and anxiety may be robbing you of perspective (when you need it the most).

"Should I stop taking my antidepressant?" There's no need to panic just because you've gotten pregnant while taking an antidepressant. One of the worst mistakes women make (sometimes, unfortunately, with their doctor's approval) is to abruptly stop taking their medication when they realize they're pregnant. Never do that. The relapse rate is extremely high, and mood disorders can hurt your baby directly and indirectly. Discuss your options with a doctor who has excellent clinical expertise in this area (see chapter 3 for suggestions on how to find a doctor). Ask his or her opinion, and determine whether slowly weaning off the medication makes sense or if you should stay on it, at least for now.

Lynda's Story

Just over three years ago I had been right in this spot, right where I was this minute, but the situation couldn't have been more different. Last time I found myself looking down at the little white stick, waiting to see if a blue line would appear. I was excited and nervous with anticipation. This time I was scared to death of the outcome, no matter whether the line appeared or not. If the line failed to show up, that probably meant that my son would be an only child forever. I had never imagined I would have only one child, but after my postpartum experience, I had started to feel that was the safest path for my family. It was amazing that even though I never wanted to experience those feelings of depression and anxiety again, I still felt a sense of disappointment that that would be my only time having a baby . . . well, that is, until I looked down and noticed the little blue line had appeared. And then I thought: What am I going to do? What are we all going to do? How am I going to do this again? Why am I doing this again? How do I fix this situation so that everything will be okay?

I have never been more scared of making a decision in my whole life. You may think: "What decision needs to be made? You are already pregnant," but that is not how I felt. My husband and I had discussed the possibility of another child many times, but our opinions on the subject varied with the day. The one thing we agreed on was that we did not want to go through the pain and torture we went through the first time. The fear of going through the postpartum depression again was so significant for us that we went on the Internet and found pregnancy clinics that performed abortions. We figured that if I never went through with the pregnancy at all, then I would never have to experience the postpartum depression again. Easy solution to a difficult problem . . . or so we thought. I called the clinic and made an appointment for that Friday at 1:00 p.m. It gave us the whole week to deliberate and figure out what we wanted to do. Every day leading up to that Friday felt like the movie Groundhog Day. *I would ask my husband, "So what do you want to do?" And he would turn to me and say, "I don't know. What do you want to do?" I felt like we were getting nowhere. A decision had to be made, and it had to be made soon, or we would lose all our options. I wanted to know what to do. I tried to reason it out with myself and come up with a list of pros and cons, but how do you reason out a decision that is mostly made up of emotions and feelings? Friday finally came, and my husband and I knew it was decision time. We talked about what it would be like if our son grew up as an only child. Some aspects of our life would be easier and some would be harder. The question we could never answer was, "Would it be better or worse for him to have a sibling?" We weighed our options and decided to have the baby. I made my husband promise that if we went through with this, he wouldn't try to convince me to stop taking my medication. He agreed, and off we rode into the sunset. Well, at least it felt that way as I stayed at work and didn't leave to attend my appointment with the clinic. I think I felt content until about 6:00 that evening. That is when the "What am I doing?" feelings started to come back.*

I guess this was my first real experience with "buyer's remorse." I felt like I had bought into something (the idea of a new baby coming into our lives) and then later wondered if I had made the completely wrong decision. Obviously my husband felt the same way, because he started asking me if I thought we had made the right decision. I honestly didn't know the answer. We had the same discussion we had earlier that day, but instead of deciding to keep the baby, we decided that it would be better for us not to have it. Since the clinic was not open on the weekend, I had to wait until Monday to make another appointment. This time the appointment was for the following day, Tuesday. When Tuesday came we found ourselves in the car heading for the clinic. I had only heard of places like this and had no idea what to expect. When we arrived at the basement office, we had to push a buzzer and wait to be let into the clinic. I figured out that that is how they keep the activists away. We were greeted by the lady at the front desk and given a stack of forms to fill out. I have never had such a hard time signing my name before. The tears were blurring my vision so much that I had no idea what I was reading. My husband was obviously second guessing this decision, too, because he turned to me and said, "Do you really want to do this?" I just looked at him and said, "I have no idea what to do." He went to the lady at the front counter and asked her if we could still change our minds during the exam and tests. She explained that we could back out at any point up until I took the pill; at that point the procedure would have already started and would need to be completed. I let the nurse take some blood when I was called into the room and waited as she confirmed that I was pregnant and that my blood levels looked good enough to continue on with the procedure. We were ushered into a quiet waiting room. This was where we waited to be called into the ultrasound room where another nurse would ensure that I wasn't having a tubal pregnancy. The tears were falling freely now . . . for both my husband and me. Were we making the right decision? How could we go through with this? As we sat and waited, the director of the clinic walked by and saw us crying. She stopped in and asked us if we would like to talk. We just started rambling on about not knowing what we should do and being so scared to go through the postpartum depression again. She calmly told us that in her experience every pregnancy is different, and if we weren't sure then we shouldn't go through with the procedure. She left us to discuss it, and that is when we were called in for the ultrasound. This time, unlike when I went to the doctor for an ultrasound with my son, the screen was turned away from me so I wouldn't see the baby. The weird part for me was that I wanted to see it. We both wanted to see it. None of this seemed real until we could actually see the little peanut that would eventually turn into a child. The nurse looked kind of surprised when I requested to see the screen, but she allowed it. The reality of the situation came crashing down on both of us. She asked if we wanted to continue forward with the procedure, and we said we weren't sure. She said that if we didn't know, then we should wait until we were sure and then come back. After she left the room, I turned to my husband and said, "If we don't do this today, then I don't want to do it ever. I don't want to come back here and deal with this ever again."

He said, "Then I think we should leave now."

"Will it be okay?" I asked.

"We will get help to get through this so we can make it okay," he answered.

After the trauma of deciding whether or not to keep the baby had passed, and along with it some of the anxiety, we still had to confront the issue of whether or not I should continue to take my medication. When dealing with the hypothetical question of whether my husband would be okay with me being pregnant and taking medication, he always answered that he would. But when the hypothetical became reality and the concerns of possibly exposing the baby to things that might cause birth defects arose, he started to waver. I knew that I needed to take the medicine. I had stopped taking it before I was pregnant with my son, and I think that contributed to the postpartum depression. I had been on it for ten years by then and found myself going through huge dips while I was off it. I did not want to have the same experience this time. Like most people of the modern age, I found myself on the computer doing searches for studies on medications while pregnant. One study I found said that the medication I was on was found to cause an increase in birth defects in rats, but only if given at forty times the maximum dosage for humans. I felt pretty good about those numbers, but my husband felt that it was still a risk that we shouldn't be willing to take. As a compromise I told him that I would make an appointment with the psychiatrist I had seen during my depression. He had over seventeen years of experience treating women with postpartum depression and had treated many women during subsequent pregnancies to prevent a recurrence. We made an appointment and waited with anticipation.

During the appointment, the doctor said that he found that without medication, the frequency of recurrence of postpartum depression was around 50 percent. Women who continued to take their medication dropped the frequency significantly. Of course, our major concern was the risk of birth defects in the baby. He said that he had not seen an increased risk in any of the women he had treated over the years; in fact, they seemed to have fewer issues during their pregnancies because they were not dealing with the depression. Finally we had found an expert who could help us make an informed decision.

We decided that it would be best for me to continue taking my medication. I needed to minimize my risk of postpartum depression and also allow myself to stay emotionally and mentally healthy during my pregnancy. I am currently ten weeks pregnant, and so far, so good. I am taking the additional measures of lining up people to stay with me and help after the baby is born so that I don't feel so isolated and alone. I think that I will be fearful about the possibility of going through the depression again until after the baby is born and I see how I react to the hormone fluctuations, but I am hoping that this time, armed with more knowledge and experience, it will be a much smoother transition for everyone.

Remember: Women at risk for postpartum depression can significantly decrease their risks by actively setting up a strategy while still pregnant.

Scenario 2: I'm on an Antidepressant (or Other Psychiatric Medication), and I Want to Get Pregnant.

"Is it ethical? What if something happens to the baby—will I be able to forgive myself?" Pregnancy is risky whether or not you're on a medication. There are never guarantees. There's a certain percentage of babies in the general population who are born with problems of various kinds, and their mothers weren't on any psychiatric medications. And there are babies born with problems whose mothers were on psychiatric medications. It's easy to jump to the conclusion that it must have been the medication that caused the problem, but be careful to avoid that faulty logic. Just because two things happen concurrently (in this case, psychiatric medication and a problem with the baby), that doesn't mean there's a cause and effect—that one caused the other to occur. In other words, most often there's no way to know if the malady would have occurred even if the woman hadn't taken the medication.

We know that untreated psychiatric disorders also are risky for the baby. Mothers who are suffering tend to receive less prenatal care, might engage in riskier behaviors (even suicide), and are more likely to use alcohol and tobacco to self-treat. Ironically, these are substances that have more serious consequences to both the mom and baby than antidepressants or other psychiatric medications. That being said, we do know that a few psychiatric medications clearly cause problems, and therefore, some medications are better than others during pregnancy. For example, lithium is preferred over valproate (also known as valproic acid, brand name Depakote) since valproate is known to cause neural tube defects in 1 to 5 percent of early first-trimester exposures.

Lithium has some risk, but it is much lower. So it is good to do your homework and speak to a practitioner who has lots of clinical experience prescribing medications for pregnant women. You're also reading this book as a responsible way to collect the best information possible so you can make good decisions about your pregnancy. So yes—it is ethical to consider pregnancy. What is not ethical is acting irresponsibly, disregarding what's in the best interest of the whole family and just doing whatever you want. You are clearly someone who cares, collects valuable information, and then determines which way to go.

You and your partner need to be clear with yourselves and each other that if medication is taken and something is wrong with the baby, no blaming will occur. Not toward yourself nor toward each other. You are doing the best job you can with the information you are gathering now, which is all any person can ask of him or herself. Even if new information comes to light, you are making the best choice you can with the information you have now. Alyse, one of my clients who was not on a medication during pregnancy, birthed a baby who was born with a leg problem. She was ready to blame herself for the issue. She convinced herself the leg problem must have been caused when, at eight weeks pregnant, she visited her sister, who was cleaning her oven with harsh chemicals. It took considerable reassurance from the pediatrician, who explained how that particular leg problem could not have been caused by oven-cleaning chemicals, before Alyse stopped punishing herself. Rebecca, another one of my clients, also not taking medication, gave birth to a baby with Down syndrome. Rebecca was plagued with the obsessive thought that she had not eaten enough green vegetables during the first trimester of pregnancy—something her family had chastised her about—and that must have been what caused the genetic defect.

So much of pregnancy is out of our control, but messages from magazines, Web sites, and other people often inaccurately give mothers-to-be the impression that there are severe consequences to even minor things they do (or don't do). The attention that pregnancy attracts can be useful, but it can also be detrimental when a woman feels constantly judged. The major priorities are that a woman makes educated and informed decisions that are tailored to her particular situation.

> You and your partner need to be clear with yourselves and each other that if medication is taken and something is wrong with the baby, no blaming will occur. Not toward yourself nor toward each other.

Paula, who needed an antidepressant due to severe depression starting in her second trimester, waited for two weeks to start taking it. She was very concerned about taking the antidepressant while she was pregnant, but she felt much better within a week and a half after starting it. Her baby was born with a collapsed lung, which inflated without intervention after two days. Paula blamed the lung issue on the antidepressant, even though there is absolutely no data connecting the two. The point is, if you're ready to blame yourself, you'll find a way, and if you decide there will be no blaming, there won't be. It's up to you. I suggest you choose the latter. It will lead to a much happier life for everyone concerned. This may sound difficult, but it *is* possible. For example, as you're making your treatment decisions, tell yourself compassionately but firmly, "I'm an excellent mom. I'm making the best decisions I can with the information I have now. That's the most anyone can expect of herself." Ideally, if you have a partner, the two of you are on the same page. If so, once you've decided which way to turn regarding a treatment plan, practice reassuring your partner. This works to help both you and your partner simultaneously. Say to each other, "We are excellent parents. These are tough decisions, and we've sought the best assistance we can. Anything can happen, with or without this treatment. If something negative happens, we've done nothing wrong. We will not fault or blame ourselves or each other. We will be able to deal with whatever comes our way."

"If I'm not able to carry a child without psychiatric medication, am I fit to be pregnant? Should I have the opportunity at all?" These questions often come from a place of self-loathing and a feeling of weakness and inadequacy. You may be thinking that since you're "weak," you should be deprived of the experience—or just that it may not be fair to the baby. Other worries may arise about whether you'll pass along the depression to your baby if it's in the genes. If you're ruminating about these questions, you may also be comparing yourself to other women who, you've decided, must be "stronger" than you are. The decision as to whether or not you're "fit" to be pregnant should be made on other bases—not whether or not you need a psychiatric medication.

Another related common worry goes like this: "The stresses and responsibilities of motherhood may cause me to relapse, so therefore I better not have a baby. I don't trust my ability to handle motherhood—I'm not strong enough."

As long as you want a baby and are committed to setting up your plan of action before the baby comes and doing what it takes to keep yourself emotionally and physically healthy, you should go forward and have a baby. Trust yourself to arrange the support you will need ahead of time, so you'll be in a good position to take care of your mommy responsibilities. You can do it. Use the affirmation, "I am taking and will continue to take good care of myself so that I'll be able to take good care of my family."

If you read through this book and decide not to get pregnant, I hope you feel good about that decision as well. The only agenda here is to help you make the right decision for you. Also, if you want a baby, remember that there are several viable ways to bring a baby into your life, and not all of them require you to be pregnant. You can still become a mother, and if you already have children, you can become a mother again without becoming pregnant. Whatever you decide, just make sure that you've chosen that for the right reasons. Make sure you're basing your decision on research, sound advice, and your own intuition about what would be right for you and your family. The wrong reasons are based on feeling weak and inadequate—like you're not good enough in some way.

This was the conclusion Jennifer and her husband came to. They very much wanted a second child, but Jennifer was hesitant to become pregnant again. She had suffered with terrible anxiety during her first pregnancy with their son, and she knew her chance of experiencing anxiety again was quite high in a subsequent pregnancy. Jennifer was adamant about not taking any psychiatric medication during pregnancy, and she didn't want to experiment with other treatments. She and her husband decided to adopt a baby girl, and that was clearly the right decision for them. Although she did go on medication due to the stresses of adoption and new motherhood, she had no qualms about taking it since she wasn't pregnant, and, as she said, "my body is mine."

SCENARIO 3: I'M PREGNANT AND I'M DEPRESSED, BUT NOT ON A MEDICATION.

"What are my choices?" You have a number of choices, and they're all good. What you need in order to feel normal may be different from what another woman needs, so what treatment(s) you end up using depends on a few factors: Your body chemistry, the severity of your symptoms, your beliefs and comfort level with various treatments, and the availability of practitioners in your area who use those treatments are some of the most important. If you're in a crisis and your depression is severe, you may need a medication to help you regain your footing. If your depression isn't severe or you'd rather use one or more of the natural and emerging treatments (see chapter 7), you can look into those. Often it's a combination of various treatments that works the best. Psychotherapy should always be included, no matter if you're using medication, nonmedical treatments, or both. Sometimes therapy alone is all it takes, with the therapist helping you to set up a practical plan of action (see chapter 9 for more details on setting up a plan for recovery) and guiding you through any uncomfortable feelings that may arise.

SCENARIO 4: I WANT TO GET PREGNANT/I AM PREGNANT, AND I'M HIGH RISK FOR DEPRESSION.

Some women who struggle with mood disorders are actually told by their physicians that they shouldn't have a baby.

I have heard this over the years mainly from my clients diagnosed with bipolar disorder. This is incorrect information that causes a lot of unnecessary grief. If you have been told that you cannot choose to have a baby due to the medication you're taking, find another doctor with more clinical experience. Please refer to the Resources section for ideas on where to find knowledgeable practitioners. One resource, the Postpartum Support International Web site (www.post partum.net), has contact information for state coordinators who may have resource lists of local doctors in your area.

If you've been diagnosed with bipolar disorder, chances are you've been prescribed a "mood stabilizer" to help keep your moods more even. There are three categories of medications that are used as mood stabilizers: lithium (a true mood stabilizer), anticonvulsants, and "atypical" or second-generation antipsychotics. As with all medications, but especially in the case of mood stabilizers, there are those that are definitely safer than others in pregnancy. And this book, along with your doctor's advice, can help you decide on your best option(s). But the point is, any woman who is capable of taking care of herself and her baby (with help) while pregnant and after the birth should be able to have a baby—no matter what the diagnosis.

> Any woman who is capable of taking care of herself and her baby (with help) while pregnant and after the birth should be able to have a baby—no matter what the diagnosis.

If you have needed medication for depression in the past, you may be feeling worried about getting pregnant again or for the first time. Consult with a psychiatrist and other support people with clinical expertise about your choices. Make sure that you, your partner, and those closest to you are clear about the warning signs of depression in pregnancy (refer to chapter 5 for a clear description of what's normal and what's not during pregnancy). Remember also that there's plenty you can do in order to prevent a recurrence, or at least greatly minimize your chances of one (see chapter 9 for a thorough plan).

Due to misinformation, women sometimes believe their choices are either not to get pregnant at all or suffer through the pregnancy without medication. This is not true. As long as you want to get pregnant, you receive proper information and support, and you're willing to follow your plan of wellness, you should go ahead. Deciding whether or not to become pregnant is an emotional decision, not one that you can decide by listing out pros and cons on a piece of paper.

Also, recognizing that you are high risk for recurrence can mobilize you and others to put together a contingency plan, so if recurrence happens, you can see your way back to wellness as quickly as possible.

How to Make the Decisions

Making any major decision can be tricky since you can be your own worst enemy by continually second-guessing yourself. Since there are no guarantees with any decision, and there are risks whether or not medication is used, for instance, it's easy to waffle back and forth with self-doubt (especially if you're depressed or anxious). "What-iffing" is what I call the activity of the worried mind conjuring up all the worst-case scenarios and possible negative consequences. Typically "what-iffing" occurs when the person has an anxiety disorder. If you're a "what-iffer," you already know who you are. One of the most common and emotionally charged "what ifs" I hear during the period of time when medication decisions are being made is, "What if I take the medication and later it's found to be unsafe in pregnancy?" You can drive yourself batty with this kind of thinking. We now know that caffeine shouldn't be ingested during pregnancy, so should those millions of mothers who drank coffee or tea or ate chocolate during pregnancy before that information came out feel guilty? Of course not.

We also know now that depression in pregnancy can hurt the baby, and researchers who specialize in the field agree that this known fact typically outweighs the possible unknown risk of taking the medication. The theory is that the chemicals released in the depressed pregnant woman cross the placenta and affect the growing baby. This is both fascinating and important information. It was once thought that if the depressed woman suffered through the pregnancy, then the baby, at least chemically, would be "safe." With this new research, however, professionals are rethinking this, and now they agree that the real danger is probably in the nonmedicating of depression in pregnancy—not in the

> Professionals agree that the real danger is probably in the nonmedicating of depression in pregnancy—not in the medicating—if medication is required for wellness.

medicating—if medication is required for wellness. ("Treatment" doesn't necessarily require medication. This research is discussed in greater detail in chapter 6.)

Some of you may recall scary stories about medications, once deemed safe, that were taken off the market due to serious side effects when taken during pregnancy. The medications around today, according to independent researchers and the most ethical of practitioners, aren't like those. There are much stricter policies these days on testing medications before they come to the public. All you can expect of yourself is to collect the most up-to-date information available and make the choices you feel are optimal based on that.

TALKING TO A PROFESSIONAL

Get all the help you feel you need when making your decisions. Professionals can be of great assistance here.

Getting Over the "Shrink" Stigma

If it feels scary to see a "shrink" for a consultation, understand that others feel that way too at first. Remember that this doesn't mean you're "crazy." Try to let go of this outdated stigma so it doesn't get in the way of you receiving the best guidance. If you needed a professional opinion about your teeth, you'd see a dentist, and the same concept applies here. You deserve the best care possible, so allow yourself to make appointments with those who have the most useful information.

The professionals you turn to should be knowledgeable and nonjudgmental. Ideally, you would work with someone who knows you well. Realistically, you may need to seek out someone with a level of expertise you might not have needed before. If you anticipate needing help, it's always best to allow a professional to get to know you before you are in crisis. Most gynecologists and psychiatrists are happy to meet with you for "preconception" appointments to discuss your options and begin a plan of action. Your partner should go with you to the doctor or therapist to receive the same information (see chapter 3 on therapy) regarding the pros and cons of various treatments. If you don't have a partner, elicit other support. If you want to see a professional alone when discussing a plan, ask yourself why as honestly as possible. If there is any sort of emotional or physical abuse or discord in the marriage or domestic situation, the professional needs to know so you both can receive the help you need. The risk of domestic abuse in pregnancy increases, probably because pregnant women are more vulnerable during this period.

Sometimes, depending on an individual's financial/health insurance situation or geographical area, expertise in pregnancy and mood disorders might be hard to find or available only in a limited way. In that case, a consultation from an expert in the field can be an extremely valuable option. Sometimes health care providers that otherwise might feel uncomfortable with treatment can help with care in a more informed way if the team includes a consultant with appropriate expertise. A consultation may be initiated by either the patient or one of the professionals on the regular care team. For instance, your OB may not feel comfortable prescribing you medication, so he might request a consultation with a psychiatrist who's known to be a specialist in prescribing to pregnant women. Often women who have a good working relationship with their regular therapists contact me (or their therapists contact me) for some specialized help with pregnancy and postpartum issues. Consultations are not ongoing; the specialist provides one assessment, with maybe a few follow-ups as needed.

DON'T BE THE ONLY JUDGE

When depression hits (or sneaks up), it's hard to make any decisions at all, let alone major ones like these. Doctors have been taken down from their pedestals, which is healthier for all concerned, including them. (Although at times it might seem appealing to have answers presented with certainty, real experts in this area know that risks and benefits of treatment options present a complicated picture. Each decision is unique and based on individual preferences and the clinical picture. Doctors can be considered as part of the team, working on your side, with you in charge.) However, those doctors—typically psychiatrists—who have excellent clinical experience treating pregnant women can be especially helpful here. The point is, especially if you're depressed, don't be the only judge when making these

> If you're depressed, don't be the only judge when making these decisions. Although ultimately the choices are up to you, trust others with the clinical experience (as opposed to just book learning) to help you.

decisions. Although ultimately the choices are up to you, trust others with the clinical experience (as opposed to just book learning) to help you. And if you're feeling well and stable, and you are making decisions now for possible treatment later in the pregnancy and postpartum, still use those in the know to help guide you.

RISKS VERSUS BENEFITS

Weighing the risks versus the benefits of using a medication during pregnancy is easier in some instances than in others. If a pregnant woman has a life-threatening bacteria that only penicillin will knock out, it's an obvious decision. But whether or not to use an antidepressant in pregnancy often feels like a gray area. Although it's improving, there's still a nasty double standard when it comes to treating other illnesses or conditions in pregnancy. It feels less clear-cut when deciding about medications for depression than, for instance, medications for treating high blood pressure or diabetes. It's important to remember that depression, too, is a life-threatening illness when inadequate treatment is received. Even during pregnancy, a certain percentage of women are so severely depressed that they attempt suicide. But even if you are not in danger of harming yourself, you need to feel well, both for your sake and for the sake of your family (including those not yet born).

There are always risks whether you take a medication or not. We take risks every day. Living is a risk.

> It's important to remember that depression, too, is a life-threatening illness when inadequate treatment is received.

Although depression and anxiety are sometimes handled without medications, if a medication is needed for you to function normally, it's responsible to decide to take it. Depression in pregnancy can hurt your baby, as chapter 9 will discuss further. Never feel guilty for needing a psychiatric medication—it does not mean that you are weak or inadequate. Rather, feel grateful that the medication is here and developed for this purpose. Don't try to tough it out—that's a mistake. You're not a failure. If a pregnant woman needs a medication to be well, whether it's a blood pressure medication or an antibiotic or an antidepressant, she should take it. It's more appropriate to treat the illness than to ignore it or to undertreat it, which can lead to chronic illness and relapse. Although professionals agree that you should take the smallest amount of psychiatric medicine as necessary during pregnancy, you should be treated to 100 percent wellness. This is true whether treatment is handled with medication and therapy, or natural treatments and therapy.

Asking the Right Questions

Bring to your appointment a list of questions to ask the OB and/or psychiatrist. If your partner or other close support person has questions, you can combine your lists into one. Ideally, your partner will be able to come with you to the appointment so he or she can hear the information at the same time.

If you've been on medications in the past, ask the pharmacist who's been filling your prescriptions if she has any suggestions for questions to ask your doctor. The pharmacist may know your medical history, what else you're taking, and possible drug interactions. *But*, keep in mind that like other health care professionals, pharmacists will differ in their knowledge and real-world experience about mental health treatment and pregnancy. Many women have been frightened by well-meaning pharmacists who tell them that it is not "safe" to take their medication if pregnant or breast-feeding. Remember to ask your doctor about any information your pharmacist mentions before stopping your medication.

Somewhere on your list you need to ask the psychiatrist if she's willing to prescribe and also monitor you throughout your pregnancy and postpartum. I should mention here that it's specifically a psychiatrist who should be managing your psychiatric medication if you in fact need it. Many OBs may prescribe an antidepressant for you, but they're typically not equipped to monitor you, and frankly, that's not their job. A psychiatrist, on the other hand, is well trained to do this. If and when you need a medication, it's important that you're not just handed a prescription, but that there's an ongoing plan to check back in, alter the dosage if necessary, and so on. However, if you cannot or will not see a psychiatrist with the recommended expertise, know that it's better to have an OB/ GYN or a general practitioner prescribe for and monitor you than to not be under anyone's care. Furthermore, it's better to be seeing a therapist and an OB/GYN or a general practitioner who are well informed about pregnancy and mood disorders than a psychiatrist who is not well educated about pregnancy and postpartum.

Inform Your Team

If you haven't needed a psychiatric medication before and therefore haven't worked with a psychiatrist, make sure your OB knows your personal and family history of mood and anxiety disorders—depression, anxiety, bipolar disorder, panic, psychosis, severe premenstrual syndrome (PMS), premenstrual dysphoric disorder (PMDD), or anything else that has affected your emotional functioning. Any of these in your past make you high risk for mood issues during pregnancy and postpartum. Don't assume that your OB knows you're high risk; make sure you give her this information. If you're not sure about the information, ask for your files to be transferred from your last doctor to your new one. And if you are high risk, make sure you get a referral to a psychiatrist just in case you need medication during your pregnancy. Even though you may be feeling great right now, it's important that the psychiatrist understands your background. He or she should know the severity of any mood disorder you've experienced, what medications you've taken for it, other treatments you've used, what treatments worked and didn't work, and the longest period of time you were able to stay off medication. If you're at risk for a mood disorder, the best plan is to create relationships with providers before you are in crisis. That way, your doctors can get to know you, your preferences and values, and plan with you for whatever might happen. And if you don't need them after all, no harm done. It will give you peace of mind knowing they're there.

If you're currently on a medication, thinking of getting pregnant, and you were able to stay off for a year or more, the psychiatrist may suggest you try to wean off your medication before you get pregnant and see what happens. On the other hand, if you tend to relapse quickly, then you'll probably be advised to stay on it. If your current antidepressant is working well for you and you need to stay on it in order to feel well, don't switch medications just because another one may have had more research done on it. This is definitely not the time to experiment. The rule is, use what works. You need to be well for your sake and your baby's sake, as well as for your marriage and other children you may already have. Again, it's not the amount of research that's thought to be the most important factor when making this decision—it's the effectiveness of the medication for you that receives the most attention.

> Don't switch medications just because another one may have had more research done on it. This is definitely not the time to experiment. The rule is, use what works.

If neither you nor a family member has ever been treated with an antidepressant, the whole smorgasbord is open to the doctor. He or she will choose one for you with an educated guess, taking both your symptoms and the research of the medication into account. If you're experiencing anxiety as a main symptom (which is very common), there are some antidepressants that tend to be more effective than others for treating it.

Medical Data versus Emotions

The factual, objective, clinical data that we have to date regarding possible risks to the baby from taking medication should be evaluated, as much as humanly possible, without emotion. It's tough enough to evaluate what's what with the medication, and that information is much more easily assimilated without the interference of personal feelings regarding taking a medication. Since the two issues—objective medical data as differentiated from feelings about taking medicine—often and easily get mixed together, I think it is important to address them individually so you can separate them out in your own mind.

Although our society is clearly going in the right direction regarding its views on taking medication for mental health, you may be worried nonetheless about the stigma of taking an antidepressant. What's most important, of course, is what you think—not what others think. If you feel that taking an antidepressant while you're pregnant will affect your self-esteem, this should be discussed with a therapist. If you're worried it will change the way you regard yourself ("What does this mean about me as a mother? How will I feel about myself?"), talk this through with a nonjudgmental professional you trust. (See chapter 3 for a discussion on finding a good therapist or discussing your feelings with a different kind of qualified professional.)

When making your decision, your individual comfort level about the possible risks associated with taking the medication should be taken into account. You need to be comfortable with whatever plan you choose and believe in the treatment plan, regardless of what combination of therapies are used. It's interesting to note that sometimes the symptoms of the illness itself—anxiety, for example—actually interfere with getting help. For instance, a woman, due to her anxiety disorder, may be too worried about taking a medication during pregnancy, and therefore she may not take something that could potentially really help her. In the context of a good psychotherapy experience, a woman may experience decreased anxiety and a safe place to discuss medication. I've found that typically, once the woman pushes through the worry and tries the medication, she's then able to more rationally evaluate the objective information and is fine with her choice since her anxiety has been quelled. I also recommend other techniques, especially Emotional Freedom Technique (EFT) or Eye Movement Desensitization and Reprocessing (EMDR) (see chapter 7 for a more in-depth description) to help with acute anxiety since these energy techniques often provide immediate relief. Sometimes EFT or EMDR is all a woman needs for her anxiety, and other times she feels relief but then still decides to take a medication. There's no wrong way. And the "right" way is the way that's right for you. Treatment is very individual.

If you're already on medication and feel anxious about continuing on it during pregnancy, you can discuss other options with knowledgeable professionals. Sometimes the anxiety is due to a lack of information, and what's needed is simply some reassurance by the doctor. If you want to explore natural methods, and the professionals with whom you're now in contact aren't aware of them or don't know enough about them to advise you, they may be able to refer you to a different type of practitioner (also see the Resources section for suggestions).

Key Points

- *Whatever you do, don't stop your medication cold-turkey if you find out you are pregnant. Pregnancy is risky whether or not you're on a medication, and untreated psychiatric disorders are also risky for the fetus.*

- *Whether you decide to take medication or not, the major priorities are that you make educated and informed decisions that are tailored to your situation.*

- *Get all the help you need when making your decisions, preferably from knowledgeable and nonjudgmental professionals.*

Chapter 2

WHEN PROFESSIONALS DON'T AGREE

As if making these important decisions isn't confusing enough, sometimes they can seem even murkier when your professional team members have conflicting points of view. This chapter is designed to help you decide whose opinion to follow when that occurs. I'll outline how, ideally, the professionals whose help you're enlisting should be cooperating, and what to do if one of them cannot or does not want to treat you. The physical and emotional risks to pregnant moms and their growing babies if medication is abruptly stopped will also be explained.

Whom Do You Listen To?

In general, medical doctors do not have much, if any, training in the area of treating mood disorders in pregnancy. This is clearly unfortunate, but it isn't their fault. Doctors are simply not taught this information in medical school. So unless they have a great deal of clinical experience (see Glossary) treating pregnant women who are depressed, anxious, bipolar, or psychotic, doctors might only be familiar with what the

Physician's Desk Reference (PDR) tells them. You've probably seen this gigantic book sitting on your doctor's desk or on her office shelf. The information in the PDR is quite limited regarding the medicines and the dosing of those medicines for pregnant women. It is often out of date or even incorrect when it comes to this specialized area. So if you ask your doctor a question about which medication might be best for you to take and see her reaching for the PDR, it's probably a safe bet that you should be seeing a different doctor (for this particular advice). This is certainly not to say that this doctor isn't excellent—she probably is. But for your specific needs at the moment, you should be working with someone who has this information at the tip of her brain, or at least knows to reach for a more sophisticated source for the information.

Most obstetricians have received little formal study on psychiatric disorders and their treatments. Many did not plan on being on the front lines with women and psychiatric disorders, but considering how common these conditions are during the reproductive years, that is indeed what they find themselves doing. Even the most well-intentioned and best-trained obstetrician will find treating psychiatric disorders challenging, based on their training, which emphasized other areas, and also their limited time per patient. The fact is, few doctors, regardless of specialty, are taught adequately during their training how to treat pregnant women with mood disorders. Since there is no treatment protocol as of yet, unless doctors attend special seminars or in-service trainings either during or after medical school, they will not have up-to-date information or sometimes any information at all on the topic. For this reason it's important that you connect with a doctor who has plenty of clinical expertise in this specialized field.

Ask your doctor for the name of a psychiatrist who has this experience, or refer to the Resources section of this book for ways to locate a knowledgeable psychiatrist. If you cannot find a doctor who has this experience, the next best idea is to locate a doctor or another professional with the ability to prescribe who has an open mind and is willing to learn. Quite often I'm contacted by wonderful M.D.s who are eager for information so they can treat their pregnant patients appropriately. I either send them medical journal references or, better yet, if they're open to it, I give them the names of M.D. specialists I know with whom they can consult. That way the professionals can speak "doctor" to each other and discuss which medications or combination of medications and doses may be best for their patients. Although OBs ask me for my opinion on this topic quite frequently, it's often best for the medical doctors to speak directly. Sometimes an OB will consult with another OB or a psychiatrist, and sometimes a psychiatrist will call another psychiatrist to bounce treatment ideas off each other. If you begin working with a psychiatrist who doesn't have the expertise and whose ego is too large to admit that he or she needs guidance from another source, change doctors.

A common situation that many pregnant women face is when one of their doctors agrees with the decision to take a particular medication and another major player disagrees. For instance, your OB may feel fine about

If you begin working with a psychiatrist who doesn't have the expertise and whose ego is too large to admit that he or she needs guidance from another source, change doctors.

prescribing an antidepressant for you in pregnancy, but the OB may instruct you to speak to the pediatrician before he will prescribe it. The pediatrician may then either discourage you or even flat out scare you by saying it would be dangerous for the baby and by no means should you take it. Now what should you do? You may be suffering from a severe depression and know you need quick help, but you don't want to do anything to hurt your baby. This situation happens, unfortunately, very frequently, and that's why I'm including this section.

Whom you listen to should definitely be based upon the professional's experience more so than the information found in books—including the PDR. Don't be impressed or swayed by the "alphabet soup" after a doctor's name, either. Many doctors with prestigious reputations and awards don't necessarily have the specific clinical expertise to help you at this juncture. Again, a particular doctor might be generally excellent, but not helpful for you in this particular situation. One of the marks of an excellent professional is when he or she acknowledges what they don't know. At that point, the doctor will typically refer you to someone else who does. I have respect for a doctor who knows her limits and doesn't expect to have all the answers. Even if it frustrates you that your doctor can't help you, it's certainly better than if she pretends she can and starts taking wild guesses instead of educated ones.

Nancy, a past client, went through this exact experience, except it was her OB who said "no" to the antidepressant and the pediatrician who said "fine." Nancy first contacted me at the end of her second trimester, at which time she was severely depressed. She was barely able to function during the day and reported just wanting to lie on her couch. She wasn't motivated to do any of her regular projects, which wasn't like her, and her self-care was poor, which also was very unlike her—she typically dressed fashionably and took pride in her appearance.

Her OB had inappropriately told her to stop her antidepressant when she suddenly found out she was pregnant. Although for a few weeks she didn't feel physically well, emotionally she felt fine for the first five weeks. Then, slowly, she started to slip down into the "pit," as she called it. This is not unusual; if a woman needs an antidepressant in pregnancy and stops taking it, the risk of relapse is quite high. (I'll discuss this in greater detail in the next section.) Nancy was afraid to call her OB since he had been so vehemently opposed to her staying on the medicine when she became pregnant. She was also feeling embarrassed for a couple of reasons. One, the depression itself made her self-esteem low, and two, she felt weak that she couldn't get through the pregnancy without needing medication. So she called me for advice. I asked her who had been prescribing the medication to her before she became pregnant, and she told me that her general practitioner (GP) had been prescribing. She then went on to tell me that when she had called the GP, he had told her that her needs were out of his realm of expertise, and she should contact a psychiatrist instead. That's the sign of a good professional, I told her. I suggested to her that she contact an area psychiatrist who specializes in prenatal and postpartum depression. This particular psychiatrist has worked with hundreds of pregnant patients, belongs to organizations that are primarily focused on the mental health of women during and after childbirth, and keeps up with the latest knowledge in the field. Nancy consulted with this psychiatrist, who agreed with the pediatrician about the safety of the medication she had been on prior and that had worked well for her. She began taking the medication, along with implementing an excellent nutrition program I recommended to her and a plan for more nighttime sleep, and she felt much better in less than two weeks.

Don't worry about hurting your doctor's feelings if you choose not to follow his advice—the doctor is there for you, not the other way around, and you know your body and your needs better than anyone.

The moral to this story is this: Please don't worry about hurting your doctor's feelings if you choose not to follow his advice—the doctor is there for you, not the other way around, and you know your body and your needs better than anyone. You are the expert of your own experience. If a doctor becomes offended and takes it personally if you listen to another professional's advice instead, you may want to find a different doctor. In fact, with complicated topics like medication use during pregnancy, many doctors will welcome a "second opinion" or team approach. It's understandable if he or she doesn't agree with your choice, but taking it personally isn't a healthy or professional response. Ego shouldn't be part of the equation. In most cases, even if the doctor doesn't agree with your decision, he or she will still work with you and help to monitor you. The doctor does, however, have a choice as to whether or not to treat you. We'll cover this later in the chapter.

Medication: Don't Just Stop

A very common and potentially dangerous mistake doctors sometimes make is to instruct their patients to immediately stop their antidepressants or other psychiatric medication when the women become pregnant. One would think there should be enough medical information published on the subject so that doctors would know better by now, but there isn't. Only those doctors with clinical experience treating mood disorders in pregnancy know this information. And, unfortunately, this phenomenon still frequently occurs

I have never met a doctor with expertise in treating pregnant women for mood disorders who would ever suggest that a patient should abruptly discontinue her medication. If an OB, GP, or PCP (primary care provider) has a patient who becomes pregnant, the doctor should quickly refer the woman to a psychiatrist (ideally she should already be working with one) who has specific expertise in this field and can determine how to proceed.

RISK OF RELAPSE
When a woman abruptly stops taking her medication, the risk of relapse is extremely high. As a matter of fact, relapse rates have been shown to be as high as 68 percent for women who stop their antidepressant when they become pregnant. Compared to 26 percent of women who become depressed even when they continue taking their medication during pregnancy, this is a substantial difference. Over 40 percent of the women who relapse start taking their antidepressants again sometime during the pregnancy. Women who have bipolar disorder are high risk for a relapse (about 70 percent) whether or not they continue their medication (usually mood stabilizers),

but their risk is much higher (about 85 percent) if they stop their meds. They also set themselves up for more recurrences and more time being ill.

Dangers to Mom and Baby

Uncomfortable and downright dangerous physical withdrawal reactions may occur for the mom—including seizures (with some classes of medication)—if psychiatric medication is abruptly discontinued. While most withdrawal reactions such as those from antidepressants are not dangerous (although they can be uncomfortable), the risk of relapse for the mom's depression is high. Also, what has occurred in the meantime when she's off her medication can jeopardize a woman's health and the health of her developing baby in numerous ways.

As mentioned before, a woman who stops her medication can emotionally crash. Sometimes this happens immediately, and sometimes it can take a few weeks as she gradually spins lower and lower. If she's bipolar, she can be catapulted into a manic episode that can be quite dangerous both for her and her baby. In a manic episode, a woman may act erratically, engaging in destructive behaviors such as using drugs, drinking alcohol, and having indiscriminate sex.

With a mood disorder that includes mania, depression, or anxiety, a pregnant woman may stop taking care of herself. She may lose her appetite and not eat, and therefore not gain enough weight. She may have insomnia and not sleep, causing worse emotional symptoms. She may not follow up with prenatal appointments at her OB's office due to lethargy, lack of motivation, or hopelessness. Plus there is a tendency for pregnant women to self-medicate when they're depressed by smoking (20.4 percent), drinking alcohol (18.8 percent), or using drugs (5.5 percent). Although many people can't fathom the idea of a pregnant woman thinking of harming herself, it happens—she may become so seriously ill that she attempts suicide.

When Deborah missed her period, she took a home pregnancy test and was surprised, yet thrilled, to find out she was pregnant. She and her fiancé, Eric, wanted children, and Eric knew from a previous marriage that his sperm count was low. They hadn't been using birth control since they believed it would be difficult to conceive. Deborah went to her OB's office to make extra sure the results were positive. When the nurse confirmed her pregnancy, Deborah noticed that the look on the nurse's face was anything but pleased. She asked Deborah to wait for the doctor before she left the office. Deborah immediately became concerned that something was wrong with the pregnancy and as she waited, she became increasingly anxious. Her OB brought her into his consultation room and, in a somber tone, inquired if she was still taking an antidepressant. She answered yes, and he then told her that he felt she should immediately discontinue her antidepressant since, he said, "the drug isn't safe for the baby." Deborah was alarmed; she had depended on the antidepressant for about three years, and it had been working beautifully for her. The OB had known she wanted children and had never mentioned the lack of safety of the antidepressant before this moment. It scared her to think of stopping the medication, but she didn't want to hurt her baby. She went home, told Eric she had to quit taking her medicine, and did just that.

It was Eric who contacted me initially. He became concerned about Deborah, who, by four months into the pregnancy, was saying things like, "I'll make a terrible mother anyway. You'll be better off with a wife who isn't defective like me. Maybe I should just leave or give this child up to a normal mother who can take care of it. I just want to die."

Eric explained that this wasn't the woman he fell in love with, and he didn't know who she was anymore. He was, as you might well imagine, upset and concerned. He couldn't console her, and she was withdrawing from him and the world more and more each day. He finally called me, he explained, "because I found her with a handful of pain medication pills. She was ready to pop them all."

Deborah didn't feel like she was worth therapy and felt it wouldn't do any good, so I suggested to Eric that he strongly request she talk with me for his sake and for the baby. She reluctantly agreed. I also gave Eric the name of a wonderful psychiatrist in their city who had the necessary background to help Deborah. Needless to say, the very next day Deborah was put back on her medication. It took about three weeks before she was completely out of the woods. She's now fully enjoying her three-month-old daughter, Emma. Deborah's story has a happy ending, but many other pregnant women aren't as lucky.

Abruptly stopping medication is also not healthy for the baby. Using the example of the scenario above, if a woman (such as Deborah) was taking a medication before she knew she was pregnant, the baby has already been exposed to the drug. When a doctor directs her to stop taking the medication, not only does the mother's body react to the severe change, but we can imagine—and this is one theory—that the baby would also experience a reaction, since the baby's body is pulled off the drug just as quickly. Then, when the mother relapses, she goes back on the medication, reintroducing the substance to the baby. That kind of on again/off again isn't ideal for anyone. There is also the added risk that the medication won't work as well for the mother again, or work quickly, leaving her ill, which is obviously not positive for her or her baby. The main point is that whatever happened in the meantime when she was relapsing and until she is re-medicated wasn't healthy for either mom or baby.

For the very few medications that pose a serious risk (for instance, valproate, which can cause neural tube defects), the risk occurs early in pregnancy, usually before a woman is even aware she is pregnant. Therefore, abrupt discontinuation of the medication makes no sense. It will only increase the risk of poor mental health but will not avoid the exposure to the baby—that's already occurred.

Do not panic if you find yourself pregnant while using psychiatric medications, and be wary of health care providers who overreact in that situation. Instead, consult someone who can advise you more soundly. Stopping "cold turkey" can lead to significant physical and emotional complications. Wait until you speak directly with a specialist in the field and receive proper guidance. Even if there's a better medication for you to take during pregnancy that could possibly replace the one you're on, you want to follow a knowledgeable professional's plan of weaning off one while substituting it with the other.

> Do not panic if you find yourself pregnant while using psychiatric medications, and be wary of health care providers who overreact in that situation.

Collaboration among Professionals

All of the professionals you're working with who are part of your wellness plan in pregnancy need to be in the loop and in agreement with the plan. Ideally, all of them are of the same opinion regarding your treatment. But even if they're not, as long as they have all accepted the plan of action, they are all informed regarding who's taking care of what, and they are all comfortable with their roles, that's all you really need. Make sure that each of your professionals has the others' contact information and that you've given each of them permission to relay pertinent information to one another. Due to recent federal laws, your professionals will probably need your permission in writing.

The professionals who will be working together on your behalf may differ from your neighbor's team of professionals. Each woman may need or want a slightly different combination of doctors and therapists. You will probably be under an OB's care, but maybe you're working with a midwife or general practitioner or some other M.D. who's overseeing your health during pregnancy. Chances are, if you've already needed to consult with a pediatrician about medication, you have him or her waiting in the wings for the big event. If you haven't already chosen a pediatrician by your third trimester, bring one on board so your baby will have a doctor lined up. To help you choose your baby's doctor, ask the potential pediatricians how comfortable they are if you choose to breastfeed while taking your medication, if you are considering that as an option. If you're already on a medication or think you may need one, a psychiatrist should ideally be involved. But, for various reasons, you might have a primary care doctor, OB, or psychiatric nurse practitioner prescribe. And, of course, you'll want a therapist as a major player. As a matter of fact, it's often the psychologist or another psychotherapist who's coordinating the professionals and keeping them informed when necessary. The reason for this is that it's the therapist who helps you identify how you're doing emotionally. Also, if you are actively involved in psychotherapy, you'll usually be seeing your therapist more frequently than your other health care providers, with the exception of the obstetrical provider at the end of pregnancy. Certainly, if you want to be the one to relay the messages back and forth, that's fine also. But when depression hits, it's easier to allow the professionals to do the orchestrating on your behalf, and it is part of their job. For that matter, even if you're feeling great emotionally, feel free to put one of your professionals in charge. It's one less job you need to handle. More often than not, I do this for my clients.

I frequently call my clients' psychiatrists to let them know what's happening with their patients emotionally. And the reverse is often true as well. For instance, the psychiatrist may call to let me know that his patient's (my client's) dosage has changed, and the doctor wants me to keep an eye out and inform him as to whether I'm seeing improvement.

One type of knowledgeable professional that is rarely mentioned when speaking of a professional team is your pharmacist. There are appropriate and inappropriate ways to utilize a pharmacist's expertise, but when done well, it can be of great help. If you have a pharmacist who's been filling your prescriptions (of anything), you might ask her to generate a list of all the medications (for everything) you're taking presently plus all the medications you've taken in the past. One way a pharmacist can assist you is by alerting you to possible negative drug interactions. If you're taking one medication, and you're thinking of asking your psychiatrist for an additional medication, the pharmacist might give you a heads-up to ask your doctor about how these two medications interact before you start taking the second.

Pharmacists are not allowed to give you medical advice, however, so be wary of that. Although pharmacists may discuss with you the risks of drugs when taken during pregnancy, by law she cannot tell you what you should take and what you should not. You can rely on your psychiatrist or another medical doctor for that advice. Remember that it's the professionals with the most clinical experience—those who have actually treated pregnant women—who you want to listen to, and pharmacists do not provide direct treatment. However, they can be a valuable part of a health care team, as pharmacists have received years of psychopharmacology training (information about how particular drugs work and possible interactions). So even though she isn't qualified to give you medical advice, your pharmacist can sometimes give you suggestions about what to ask your doctor. She may also know your history, other medications you've been on, and personal drug reactions, and she is often willing to speak directly to your M.D. regarding your situation.

If a Doctor Refuses to Treat You

Although unusual, it sometimes happens that a psychiatrist or other medical doctor will refuse to treat a pregnant patient if she decides to use a psychiatric medication while pregnant. If you run into this situation, please don't take it personally. This isn't a statement about you or your judgment. Doctors make this decision for one of two major reasons. The first reason is that he doesn't have the expertise necessary to treat and monitor you. He may completely agree with your need to be on the medication, but he's acknowledging that this area is beyond his know-how. This simply means that you will need to find a doctor who has the necessary background. Unbelievably, just a few years ago, psychiatrists were still being taught the myth that reproductive hormones protected women from mood disorders in pregnancy, so medication was not necessary. Therefore, the old thinking was that doctors didn't need to learn how to prescribe psychiatric medication for pregnant women.

The second reason is that some doctors just aren't willing to treat pregnant women with psychiatric medication. The doctors may have the knowledge, but they don't want to risk being held liable in case a parent sues if there's a problem with the baby. This makes no sense to me whatsoever. If anything, I think the opposite might start happening— lawsuits might be filed if a doctor refuses to treat a patient when she needs help. Here's why the doctor's reasoning is faulty. With any other condition that poses a large health risk to the mother and the baby, like high blood pressure, for instance, the doctor would of course treat it. This is an interesting phenomenon, since there is much more research regarding the use of psychiatric medication in pregnancy than research for medications to treat high blood pressure in pregnancy. In any case, whether it's the first reason, the second, or a combination of the two, it's good news. It's better that you know now so you can get on with the task of finding someone more appropriate for your needs.

A referral from someone you trust is always the best place to start when it comes to finding an excellent doctor—whether it be a psychiatrist or an OB/GYN. If you know someone in your situation who's had a good experience with a particular doctor, that would be a good bet. Also, a therapist in your geographic area who specializes in treating pregnant or postpartum women with mood disorders will probably know at least one psychiatrist who can help you. Another idea is to go to Postpartum Support International's Web site (www.post partum.net), which lists state coordinators. If you contact the coordinator from the state in which you live, she can often direct you to more local resources. Refer to the Resources section at the back of this book for more suggestions.

Key Points

- *Most M.D.s don't have much training in treating mood disorders during pregnancy, so it is important that you connect with a specialist in the field.*

- *Don't be swayed by the "alphabet soup" after a doctor's name—when making medication decisions, listen to the professionals with the most clinical experience, and don't hesitate to seek a second opinion.*

- *As part of your wellness plan, surround yourself with a team of professionals and make sure they are all kept in the loop about (and are accepting of) your treatment plan.*

- *A referral from someone you trust is always the best place to start when looking for a new doctor.*

Chapter 3

THE IMPORTANCE OF THERAPY

Although it's great news that medical doctors are now recognizing that mood disorders occur in pregnancy and that medication is sometimes required, it's also important that therapy is prescribed along with the meds. This is especially important for the treatment of depression during pregnancy, since this is a time that involves a major life transition into parenthood. There are many different types of therapy, but this chapter will concentrate on the talk therapy kind—the sort of therapy that involves speaking with a psychotherapist. There are even different types of talk therapy, and I'll outline a few of the most common. That way, if you have a preference, you can ask the therapist which type she usually practices. The benefits of talking through your situation with a therapist (or another wonderful professional you trust) will be discussed in depth here, and I'll also provide you with simple guidelines for choosing a therapist.

Pills Are Not Enough

In our society especially, there's a rampant notion that all one needs to do to fix an ailment is pop a pill. Although a pill may be part of the solution when it comes to alleviating a mood disorder, it should never be regarded as the entire answer for recovery. You may be disappointed to learn this, since it's so simple to think that all you need is something out of a bottle to make the emotional pain go away. Particularly when it may have taken a while for you to decide to use the medication in the first place, it's only natural that you would want it to make all your problems float away quickly and thoroughly. However, even when a mood disorder is mainly (or completely) caused by biochemical changes in the body, some processing of the feelings and thoughts that accompany mood disorders is important for a solid and lasting recovery.

My client Janet experienced a postpartum depression with her second child, and she took an antidepressant that helped her. At that time, she confessed to me when she contacted me recently, she hadn't wanted to speak with a therapist since she was afraid her friends would laugh at her and think she was "weird." This time, in her third pregnancy, the depression didn't wait until after the baby was born: She began feeling depressed in her second trimester. Scared that she was already going downhill, she called me. I remember how confused she sounded when she first called—a very common phenomenon. She asked, "Dr. Bennett, can postpartum depression start *before* the baby is born? Is that possible?" I explained to her how common prenatal depression is, and that she's in good company. I also told her how common it is for a depression to start earlier with the next pregnancy. Since Janet had not been in therapy during her bout of postpartum depression a few years ago, she didn't have a plan of action. She also hadn't had the benefit of solid information about what her brain chemistry was doing or techniques to handle her worries and roller-coaster moods. She now is set with a great plan of action, and she is being evaluated by the psychiatrist who helped her last time, so that a strategy for medication—either during the pregnancy, after the birth, or both—will be discussed.

It's wonderful that medical doctors of all kinds are now recognizing that mood disorders in pregnancy are real and need treatment. That certainly wasn't the case a few years ago. However, it's not good when a doctor simply hands a woman a prescription for psychiatric medication without also suggesting that she speak to a therapist or increase her support in some way. That should never occur. When a doctor prescribes a medication for a mood disorder, that prescription should usually be accompanied by a referral to a therapist. If for some reason this is not possible, other ways to increase your support should be discussed. Peer support groups and parenting support groups, for instance, are two ways you can increase your support.

> When a doctor prescribes a medication for a mood disorder, that prescription should usually be accompanied by a referral to a therapist.

Common Types of Therapists

You will probably have your choice of different types of therapists to talk with. What's most important—even more so than the person's credentials—is who the person is, how open she is to learning about your situation, her level of compassion, and her ability to help you. Whether your goal is to recover from a mood disorder in pregnancy, discuss a plan to help you postpartum, explore your feelings about being high risk, or anything else, it's important that you feel comfortable with the therapist and her expertise. The following is a list and short description of some of the most common types of therapists who may be of help to you now or later, including clinical psychologists, psychiatrists, marriage and family therapists, social workers, psychiatric nurses, and counselors.

- **Clinical psychologists** *focus on the diagnosis, treatment, and prevention of all mental and emotional disorders. They have earned a doctorate-level degree (either a Ph.D. or a Psy.D.), which reflects the longest period of training for psychotherapists. Clinical psychologists cannot prescribe medication, but they've received extensive training in assessment, research, and the use of various kinds of therapies.*

- **Psychiatrists** *are medical doctors who have had at least four years of special training on top of what was required to receive their medical degree. Psychiatrists are trained in psychotherapy and have been schooled in psychiatric diagnoses, psychopharmacology, and the prescribing and monitoring of medications for their patients. They are the best professionals to consult if you need a psychiatric medication. Not all psychiatrists are equally knowledgeable about prescribing in pregnancy, however, so* *you need to inquire whether the doctor is willing and able to prescribe to you if you need a medication at that time.*

- **Marriage and family therapists** *have a master's-level license (M.F.T.) and are trained in individual, couples, and family therapy. They cannot prescribe medication, but they can be a good resource if you are working through issues in your marriage that are adding to your concerns about becoming pregnant or dealing with depression/anxiety in pregnancy.*

- **Social workers** *have a master's degree—usually a master's in social work (M.S.W.)—or are licensed clinical social workers (L.C.S.W.s). Social workers are trained to understand social and environmental issues and the impact of these factors on mental and emotional disorders. Many are also trained in psychotherapy.*

- **Psychiatric nurses** *have an A.P.R.N. (advanced practice registered nurse) license. They're registered nurses who have additional training and have obtained the equivalent of a master's (and sometimes a doctoral) degree. Usually they can provide full psychiatric care under the supervision of a physician. Depending on the state in which they practice, they might also have the authority to prescribe medication.*

- **Counselors** *are master's-level mental-health professionals who have L.C.P.C. (licensed* *clinical professional counselor) licenses. They cannot prescribe medication.*

OTHERS IN THE HELPING PROFESSIONS

There are other kinds of professionals within the helping professions who may be of use to you during this time. They should never practice therapy since doing so is against the law (they're not licensed as psychotherapists), but, especially when you can't find one of the previously mentioned therapists, these professionals may provide support and compassion, and can help you consider other resources for your general well-being:

- **A certified midwife,** *educated in the field of midwifery and certified by the American College of Nurse-Midwives, is able to provide primary health care to women, including prenatal care, gynecological exams, and care during labor and delivery. They can also provide care for you and your baby postpartum. Your midwife can be a great support to you as you're trying to find an appropriate therapist or counselor.*

- **A certified birth doula** *(pronounced "doolah") supports the mother through labor and delivery, and sometimes postpartum as well. Having this type of emotional support during labor and delivery can cut the rate and severity of postpartum mood disorders. Studies show that women who are supported by a doula are less depressed, less anxious, and have higher self-*

esteem and more self-confidence after delivery than those who haven't used a doula. **Post-partum doulas** *take care of the new mom in numerous ways and can remain to help for many weeks following the delivery. They provide added emotional and physical support, education, and other help with the challenges of being a new mom.*

- **Pastoral counselors,** *who are members of the clergy (such as priests, rabbis, and ministers), often have both training and experience in mental-health issues since members of their congregations frequently seek their advice. Counselors who are open-minded, knowledgeable, and compassionate may be of great comfort to you, and often they attempt to help you find a more appropriate therapist.*

Choosing a Therapist

If you have a mood disorder and are taking a medication, or using any other treatment method for that matter, you should also be talking to a clinical psychologist or another type of licensed psychotherapist. If you do not have a mood disorder but you know you're high risk and want to be proactive, this section is for you, too. Soaking in this information in case you need it will give you the peace of mind you're seeking. Even if you've been taking a medication for a while and are feeling good, checking in with a therapist periodically during your pregnancy is a smart thing to do. When you near your due date, you might want to increase the frequency of your appointments with the therapist since she can help monitor you and make sure you have a solid plan of action for after the baby comes.

There are additional ways in which a therapist can be of support to you now. For example, it helps tremendously to have someone who is able to objectively monitor your moods. Sometimes we are able to self-monitor our moods, but often by the time women realize they are in the midst of a full-blown depression, it's too late. Moods can be confusing during pregnancy in general, and particularly when a mood disorder is present. Sometimes the psychiatrist explains this, but if not, your therapist should be able to. Also, it is comforting to discuss with and get help from a professional regarding how the mood issues may be affecting different aspects of your life: your job, your relationships, your ability to function, your changing roles and responsibilities, plus whatever concerns you might have. The point is, medication should not be used instead of therapy—it is not a substitute. Research clearly shows that therapy in combination with medication is more effective than just medication used alone.

> Research clearly shows that therapy in combination with medication is more effective than just medication used alone.

Sometimes psychiatrists provide therapy (usually the long-term kind) as well as prescribe medication, and sometimes they just take care of the medication aspect. So if you're seeing a psychiatrist just for medication management, make sure you find a qualified therapist who, hopefully, specializes in prenatal and postpartum mood disorders. A good psychiatrist will also provide support and take the time to understand what is happening in your life and with your moods, even if they are not technically providing psychotherapy. Providing medication without this support is not sufficient on their end.

If your mood disorder didn't begin during pregnancy, you'll probably find that it feels different while you are pregnant. Mood disorders in pregnancy and postpartum, especially depression, feel different than those occurring at other times in your life. The main reason for this, professionals believe, is because your hormones are involved in ways that they're not at other times. Therapists who have specific training in the perinatal mood disorders (mood disorders occurring during pregnancy and postpartum) understand how these symptoms may present themselves during pregnancy. The specialist will also understand the particular worries and stressors you may be facing during pregnancy that wouldn't necessarily be present otherwise. Specific physiological changes, psychological changes, and issues such as sleep deprivation, demands of parenting, and role changes do not collide at other times like they do during pregnancy and postpartum.

> Mood disorders in pregnancy and postpartum, especially depression, feel different than those occurring at other times in your life.

GUIDELINES FOR CHOOSING A THERAPIST

No matter whom you're speaking with—a psychologist, marriage and family therapist, or other professional—the quality of your life should be moving forward, and you should feel that you're truly receiving the help you need. This person should not be someone who tells you what to do, but someone who can help you figure out a plan that you feel good about. Being pregnant can be challenging enough without depression or anxiety (or the fear of a mood disorder happening).

There are a few ways to judge whether or not you've found someone who may really assist you. For one, if you're depressed, your mentor should help you understand that you are not your depression (or anxiety, and so on)—it's just something you need to deal with at the moment.

Psychotherapists vary in approach and methods. Some psychotherapists encourage patients to spend a great deal of time discussing their childhood without moving forward to their lives in the present. For some situations time may not be of the essence, but when a woman is pregnant and a baby's arrival is impending, she needs relief as quickly as possible. Goals of therapy should be focused on increasing your support and empowerment. Therapy should feel safe but move you forward. It may be somewhat challenging as you learn better ways of coping and improving your life while always feeling safe. After all, what feels "safe" is what's familiar—but that doesn't mean it's healthy. A talented therapist can nudge you out of your "comfort zone" in the unhealthy, familiar patterns and into a much healthier (although new and unfamiliar, at first) place. If after a few weeks you do not feel your life is moving in a positive direction, and feel you do not have trust in your therapist, you might want to change therapists.

The point is, you deserve better, so work with someone who is positive, uplifts and empowers you, helps you feel hopeful, challenges you to face your problems in a constructive way, and helps you avoid repeating patterns of behavior that haven't worked for you. This will enable you to maintain perspective as you make your important decisions, allowing you to understand that this too shall pass and will lead to happier times.

In the Resources section, you'll find http://postpartum.net, the Web site for the organization Postpartum Support International (PSI). You can find the coordinator for your state and contact her. She may be able to suggest therapists in your area. This does not automatically make them good therapists or qualified therapists, but it's a good place to begin if you haven't received a referral yet. You should still interview the therapists you're referred to through PSI or through any other source to find out if they're qualified to work with you and if the "chemistry" is good between the two of you. Make sure your therapist is credentialed, appropriately educated, and maintains professional boundaries (for instance, she doesn't call you and invite you out to lunch socially). Steer clear of a professional of any kind who does not accept that mood disorders are real disorders.

Here are four of the most important questions to ask when you're checking out therapists:

1. "Which organizations that you belong to specifically focus on mood disorders in pregnancy and postpartum?"

If a therapist says she specializes in mood disorders in pregnancy and/or postpartum, you should expect that she would belong to at least one organization devoted to this specialization.

2. "Which books and Web sites specifically focused on mood disorders in pregnancy and postpartum do you recommend?"

As with any other specialty, the therapist should be able to rattle off a few books and Web sites that focus on this area.

3. "Where have you received your specific training in mood disorders during pregnancy and postpartum, and how many hours have you completed?"

Some therapists surprisingly assume that one afternoon of training is enough to qualify them as a specialist. This is not only silly, it could be dangerous for the women they're treating. The professional should be regularly attending conferences where there are one- and two-day trainings. Some of the best trainings are the official Postpartum Support International classes that are presented around the country by trained educators. I helped to develop the curriculum for that training and taught the classes for PSI for many years.

4. "About how many women have you helped who were facing mood disorders specifically during pregnancy and postpartum?"

If the therapist answers this question by explaining that she has worked with many depressed women (but not pregnant ones) and it's all the same, call someone else. Or if the therapist has only worked with a handful of pregnant women with mood disorders, you may or may not want to be one of her first clients.

If the therapist cannot answer these questions with ease, thoroughness, and confidence, move on to another.

UTILIZING A SPECIALIST

I'm often called by women whose regular therapists have suggested that they receive some specialized help. Their therapists correctly realize that at least some of the help that their clients need is beyond their expertise. There are various ways to utilize a specialist. One, you can temporarily leave your regular therapist and start working with the specialist until after the postpartum period. Two, you can alternate one week with your regular therapist and the next with the specialist. Three, you can intersperse a few "specialized" sessions here and there as needed. Sometimes only one or two of these sessions is all that's needed before returning to the regular therapist.

STILL NOT SURE ABOUT THERAPY?

I hope you are open to finding a wonderful therapist to help you make your decisions and to see you through whatever you're facing right now. If, by any chance, you are concerned about attending therapy due to the old and weakening stigma of seeing a therapist, I'd love to convince you in the kindest of ways to get over it. It's important that you take the steps that will help you the most, regardless of what you're afraid someone else will think. However, if you are still opposed to working with a licensed therapist, you have options.

Life Coaches

Life coaches are increasing in popularity, so I want to give you this word of warning. Sometimes those who are worried about speaking to a psychotherapist due to a fear of being stigmatized feel more comfortable seeking the assistance of a life coach, but caution should be taken. Although there are exceptions to what I'm about to say (and I know some of these wonderful people personally), I definitely do not recommend that you work with a life coach regarding a mood disorder—not if you're in the middle of one or even planning in case of the possibility of one. The excellent life coaches I know agree with me completely. When a woman calls them, clearly suffering from depression, for instance, they responsibly refer her to a health care professional. But most life coaches won't be able to assess when they're "hearing" a mood disorder like my friends can. Anyone can call him- or herself a "life coach"—there is no particular expertise or qualifications that one needs to have, so basically, you have no idea where your guidance is "coming from" or what it's based upon. If you're determined to work with a life coach, then I recommend that you at least go through the International Coaching Federation (ICF) at www.coachfederation.org. This Web site provides a search tool to help you find a credentialed coach. "Credentialed" does not mean they are licensed professionals, so again, be careful.

Another type of mentor, such as someone in the clergy, who has your best interest at heart and is nonjudgmental would be your next choice. It's not generally a good idea to put a family member (even a family member who's a mental-health professional) in this role as it's difficult to impossible for him or her to keep emotions out of the picture. You need someone who can be objective and isn't invested emotionally in the outcome of whatever you decide. Remember that professionals who are not licensed therapists may not legally provide therapy, but it may still be very therapeutic to speak with them.

Whomever you choose to work with, your decision should be based more on the person's expertise, belief system, character, knowledge about your particular situation, and ability to help you than about the credentials following her name. No matter what, you need and deserve to be talking about what's happening with someone with whom you're syntonic (have good chemistry with), comfortable, and "click" with so you can set up a plan of action that will help you move forward.

A support group can be wonderful, but it is not a replacement for individual therapy. If you're thinking, "all I need is to talk to other women who are going through the same thing," that's wishful thinking. Sometimes this may suffice if you're in a mild episode or just want to "plug into" a support network just in case you need it later, but if you're experiencing a moderate to severe mood disorder, a support group, while helpful, is only one piece of your plan—you still need an individual plan of recovery just for you.

Types of Talk Therapy

The talk therapies most frequently practiced that have been shown to be effective with mood disorders in pregnancy and postpartum (and generally) are Cognitive-Behavioral Therapy (CBT) and Interpersonal Therapy (IPT). There are others that show great promise as well, such as Dialectical Behavior Therapy or DBT. (For more information on DBT, look at Susan Dowd Stone's contribution to *Cognitive Behavior Therapy*, edited by Ranen and Freeman.) I'll briefly describe each of these therapies later in this section. All of them are considered to be short-term therapies as opposed to long term, although DBT is usually a longer process than the other two. The most common long-term therapy is psychoanalysis, whereby the therapist focuses mainly on the early childhood experiences of the client. The underlying concept here is that these early memories are at the root of what's occurring now. The belief is that there's a need to understand the unconscious mind and receive insight into the past in order to move forward with one's life in the present.

There are different types of psychotherapy, representing different schools of thought. However, some are meant to be long term and some short term. For a pregnant or postpartum woman with depression, it is urgent that she feel better as soon as possible for her own sake and for her family, so short-term, goal-directed therapies make sense for her at this time. Psychoanalysis is an intensive, long-term treatment that many people might find useful, but it is not an appropriate treatment for serious mood disorders during pregnancy and postpartum. Some psychodynamic techniques (that might help a woman understand why she is feeling a certain way) might be useful, but in the context of a therapy that is meant to bring relief sooner rather than later. The crisis needs resolving first before long-term therapy should even be considered. As my friend and mentor Dr. Susan Hickman always said, "When a house is on fire, you put the fire out first before rewiring the house!"

I am a strong believer in solution-focused, short-term therapies because I've seen the kinds of benefits they effect in the lives of pregnant and postpartum women who are suffering. One of the purposes of an effective therapy is something called psycho-education, which is when the therapist provides clear information to the client that will support the goals of therapy. Research has shown that the more a person is aware of her illness and how it affects her own life and others' lives around her, the more control that person has over her illness. This means that, with appropriate knowledge and techniques, episodes of mental illness occur less often and are usually less severe and don't last as long. What's happening in the here and now is the focus—dealing with what is getting in the way of your enjoyment of life at this moment. This includes your fears, worries, ways of thinking, environmental barriers, difficulty with relationships, roles, and whatever else you may experience as a hurdle to feeling happy. If an issue from childhood happens to rear its head and need attention in order for you to make progress, it's dealt with only when and if that's the case.

Therapy is a necessary piece of your wellness puzzle, and it doesn't necessarily need to last a long time. You deserve to understand what is happening with your body and in your mind, and working with an excellent professional can facilitate that tremendously. Can you feel better without therapy? The answer is typically "yes"; however, it can take much longer, and depression can more easily come back to haunt you later in your life. Therapy works as a recovery tool, plus it's an ounce of prevention that's well worth it to help ensure your future happiness.

There are many different excellent types of therapy. Some therapists use one and only one type quite strictly, and others may have their favorite methods but use more than one. Some of the best therapists use this eclectic approach—that is, they pick and choose from among the best of the methods. Rather than rigidly sticking with one type of therapy no matter what, these therapists deftly move in and out of various therapies and techniques depending upon what each client needs at any particular time.

Not all of the types of therapy have been researched regarding their efficacy with helping depression in pregnancy, but Cognitive-Behavioral Therapy (CBT) and Interpersonal Therapy (IPT) are two that have. Please remember that more is involved in the effectiveness of therapy than just the type of therapy. For instance, as discussed earlier in this chapter, the rapport between you and your therapist can make a big difference in the outcome.

A third type of therapy I want to mention is Dialectical Behavior Therapy (DBT). There isn't, as of yet, research on this one regarding the helpfulness with pregnant women who are experiencing mood disorders or preventing mood disorders in high-risk women. However, anecdotally speaking, the therapists I know who mainly use DBT and the pregnant women who experience it are quite positive about its success.

COGNITIVE-BEHAVIORAL THERAPY

Cognitive-Behavioral Therapy (CBT) focuses on helping you change distorted, unrealistic, and negative thinking to healthy, realistic, positive thinking. Negative thoughts you have about yourself and repeat often lead to bad feelings and low moods, and enough of it can lead to depression. This pattern can be turned around with CBT techniques. Changing your thoughts can change your moods and lead you out of depression into a happier life.

INTERPERSONAL THERAPY

Interpersonal Therapy (IPT) is a time-limited, problem-oriented type of therapy that focuses on role changes in your life. The purpose of IPT is to strengthen your relationships and your ability to communicate. There have been studies indicating that IPT can be an effective nonmedical treatment for some depressed pregnant women; however, some women will need a combination of IPT and medication to be well. Research also shows that IPT may help prevent postpartum depression when used with pregnant women who are high risk.

DIALECTICAL BEHAVIOR THERAPY

Dialectical Behavior Therapy (DBT) utilizes some of the same techniques as CBT, but it also incorporates the practice of mindfulness (nonjudgmental awareness moment to moment). The most serious issues are handled first by the therapist, and the levels of problems are resolved in stages. Both individual therapy and group therapy must be used, and telephone support from the therapist in between sessions occurs as well. This theory states that some people, due to invalidating environments in their past and due to biological factors, react abnormally to emotional stimulation. DBT is a method of teaching skills that will help them cope more effectively.

Key Points

- *Therapy is a necessary piece of your wellness puzzle.*

- *Although medication may be a part of your treatment plan, pills by themselves are not enough.*

- *If at all possible, find a therapist who specializes in perinatal mood disorders.*

- *The talk therapies most frequently practiced that have been shown to be effective with mood disorders in pregnancy and postpartum are Cognitive-Behavioral Therapy (CBT) and Interpersonal Therapy (IPT).*

Chapter 4

TRUST YOURSELF

Whatever you call it—intuition, your inner voice, God, your higher self, your gut feeling, spirit guide, or angel—listen to it and trust it. You know exactly what I'm talking about, and each person experiences it in a unique way. But you know what it feels like or sounds like to you. While you were growing up, you may have been taught by the adults around you to ignore it. You may also have been taught to stay in your intellectual head, so to speak, instead of tuning in to what felt right. Or you may have been instructed to value only what others said to be true—parents, other authority figures in your life, or the media. Regarding your current situation, although it's wise to seek advice and information from professionals who practice in the field, in the end, please trust yourself. You deserve to feel good about your choices. This chapter provides you with examples of how to respond to insensitive or critical people. At the end of the chapter, you'll also see suggestions about what to do when your partner or doctor doesn't agree with your decision about medication.

Vulnerability

Some people, including some medical and mental-health professionals, still think that pregnancy protects women from illness—both physical and mental. This couldn't be further from the truth. Pregnancy is a vulnerable time for women both physically and emotionally, even when there aren't especially tough decisions to make. Pregnancy actually compromises the immune system, which makes catching colds and other viruses easier than ever. That's one of the reasons why excellent nutrition during pregnancy is key (see chapter 8 for a complete discussion on nutrition). Major hormonal changes render pregnant women very vulnerable to mood disorders as well. One in seven (15 percent) pregnant women is clinically depressed.

> **One in seven (15 percent) pregnant women is clinically depressed.**

Even without depression or anxiety, you may feel more sensitive than usual. Pregnant women are often surprised at their larger-than-life responses to statements and events that usually aren't even on their radar. For instance, the silly comments that Marissa's husband had always made about their dog never bothered her before. She could let the statements roll off her back and even found them funny at times. But when she was pregnant, she became easily annoyed by those very same comments, which surprised both her and her husband. It is quite common to be more sensitive emotionally when pregnant.

To add insult to injury, this sensitivity is even more heightened since, when you're pregnant, it seems like everyone feels entitled to tell you their opinions about anything and everything related to pregnancy and child rearing. Whether the subject is exercise, weight gain, how you'll feed your baby, or where the baby will sleep, many people you meet will dump their bias on top of you whether you're interested in hearing it or not. Even your emotions will be scrutinized. I remember a coworker asking me in my first trimester if I was filled with awe about my baby. I could tell he was bursting with information he wanted to "share" with me. I opened up a bit and explained to him that my husband and I were both carriers of Tay Sachs disease, which meant that our baby had a 25 percent (one in four) chance of having this recessive gene disorder. There isn't a cure yet for Tay Sachs, and it's 100 percent fatal. I knew I would need an amniocentesis at four months, and it would take six full weeks for the results, unlike the usual ten days. When I told him, "No, I'm not getting excited yet since I don't know if my baby's okay," he was offended and shocked. There wasn't a glimmer of understanding or compassion— only judgment. "Well," he smirked, "my wife was elated right from the beginning, and that's how it ought to be." That was over twenty-four years ago, and I still remember his disapproving look, complete with eyebrows raised. It's interesting the way those instances seem to become indelibly etched in the brain when sensitivity is high.

The myth of the happy, glowing pregnant woman filled with eager anticipation still hangs around today. Now, don't get me wrong. Some women certainly do in fact glow with happy anticipation (as opposed to the flush caused by nausea)! However, there are many—maybe you're among them— who are dealing with anxiety, depression, or other mood issues, or are worrying that they may be hit with mood problems later on. Sometimes there are external situations causing the mood discomfort, and sometimes it's due strictly to the biochemical changes of the pregnancy. At other times it can be a combination.

For example, Suzanne was having moderately anxious thoughts during the first few weeks of pregnancy. The thoughts were annoying and sometimes disturbing because of their content, but they generally didn't get in the way of her day. She didn't feel entirely steady, but she was able to function pretty well. That was, until she received lab results that indicated she had gestational diabetes. She had been teetering on the edge of severe anxiety, and the negative health news tipped her over that edge. Suzanne began having panic attacks, and that's when she called me.

Another client, Maggie, had been dealing very effectively with a mild depression in her pregnancy. She was trying to stay off medication, and I had suggested that she look into two separate alternative treatments. She began using a light box every day for phototherapy (see chapter 7) and she also began a special nutritional program (see chapter 8), each of which had made an obvious positive difference for her both emotionally and physically. Her mild depression was on its way out, and she was quite happy and hopeful. Her appointments with me were spread out to once a month. When her husband, Ed, announced in her third trimester that he was being immediately transferred by his company to Arizona (they lived in New Jersey), Maggie lost some of her footing. That kind of abrupt change would be difficult for many people, and when it happens in pregnancy, an extremely vulnerable time, negative repercussions are common. Maggie's whole support system was on the East Coast. The thought of leaving her mother, with whom she was very close and who was also the person who was going to watch the baby when she went back to work, was very sad and also scary. In two days, Maggie went from feeling good to feeling down and also shaky with anxiety. The sadness was in the normal range considering what she was facing, so good old talk therapy handled that. But the anxiety was mainly at night, giving her insomnia. A relaxation tape helped her slightly, but not enough. This occurred before I started working with some wonderful researchers who have developed a completely safe method to help insomnia (see chapter 7), so Maggie asked her general practitioner for a small dose of antianxiety medication just to help her relax and sleep at night. That was all she needed. The nutritional system and the phototherapy were still enough to keep the clinical depression at bay, but Maggie intelligently increased the frequency of her therapy appointments. She is now three months postpartum and is doing great, continuing with counseling, her nutrition, and the phototherapy.

(Just a note—if at all possible, when you're pregnant it is not the right time to move, add on to your house, change jobs, or make any other big changes. Try to plan accordingly and avoid major upheavals during that time. In chapter 5, I'll discuss why this is so important to remember.)

Along with the vulnerability experienced in pregnancy often comes a feeling of self-doubt. Another client, Mindy, expressed disgust and impatience as she described her pregnant self as "wimpy" and having "no backbone." Mindy exclaimed during a recent session, "This isn't the real me! Mindy Peters can stand up to anyone—I'm strong. Right now, I feel like a spineless lump. I have to keep asking other people what I should do. Then, after I make the decision I'm not sure it was the right one. Ridiculous!" Depression and anxiety steal away self-confidence. But even without a clinical

> Hormonal changes, the new life experience of being pregnant, and worry about trying to do everything "right" and perfect for the baby can all contribute to uncertainty.

mood disorder, as in Mindy's case, many pregnant women experience this uncertainty about their actions and decisions. This can happen for a variety of reasons: Hormonal changes, the new life experience of being pregnant, and/or the woman's worry about trying to do everything "right" and perfect for the baby can all contribute to uncertainty.

So if it's challenging just deciding what to eat for breakfast, imagine how difficult it is dealing with judgmental people saying things like, "how could you risk your baby's health by taking a medication?" If you are already taking a medication (or are thinking about taking one), that was a major decision, and you may have debated for a while. If you're feeling unsure or vulnerable to comments like these, you need to become very clear in your own mind that you made the best decision you could, and the one that was right for you. Then you can feel good about it and stop doubting yourself. Here are some tips on how to handle these comments.

First, don't take it personally and get your feelings hurt, and don't become defensive and feel like you need to strike back harshly in order to protect yourself. Remember that comments like the example I gave above come from ignorance. It has nothing to do with you. Someone who would confront you like that is a critical person in general—he or she says offensive things like this to everyone. It comes from a high and mighty attitude, from a know-it-all point of view. Of course, the more secure you feel about your decision, the easier it will be to handle these situations. The calmer you are on the inside, the more in control you'll feel. You have some choices as to how to respond, and I'll propose a couple of them. Depending on the situation, you can ignore the rude comment and walk away. Or you can answer like this: "I used to think the same thing until I did my homework and found out that I'd be risking my baby's health even more if I did *not* take the medicine. Depression crosses the placenta." That usually shuts them up.

One client of mine, Carole, had to deal with comments like this from her father-in-law, a medical doctor who is a general practitioner (GP). Although he's a nice guy who means well, "he has an ego as large as my state of Texas," Carole lamented. When he found out that Carole and her husband, Peter, had decided that Carole would start taking an antidepressant in her third trimester to help prevent postpartum depression, he put on his most authoritative voice and told them that their decision wasn't smart. Peter looked his father in the eye and said, "All the specialists in the field disagree with you, Dad. We love you, but we're listening to them." Carole said that Peter's father quietly grumbled a couple of times under his breath, and then he dropped it. His son had respectfully but firmly put him in his place.

With most people, you can avoid the conversation completely. They don't need to know about any of these major decisions you're making. The general rule is, don't share any information, especially about topics you're vulnerable about, with anyone who you're not absolutely sure will support you. (We'll talk about how to handle it if your partner doesn't support your decision a bit later in this chapter.) Protect yourself, and avoid those situations whenever possible.

Kathy's Story

My experience with postpartum depression started a couple weeks after I had my son. I wasn't sure what exactly I was experiencing; I just knew something didn't feel right. I tried to ignore my symptoms, but they just wouldn't go away. Exhausted, I felt like such a failure because I was having a hard time adjusting to being a mom. I would also have horrible thoughts of something happening to the baby, which would make me feel crazy for having the thoughts in the first place. So when my baby was about three months old, I finally got help and saw a postpartum depression therapist, Dr. Shoshana Bennett, who was so wonderful and understanding. I couldn't believe that other women felt this way, too. So I found out the reason I was having the horrifying thoughts about my son was because I have obsessive compulsive disorder. Now since I knew what it was, I thought I was all better, but I was wrong. I started taking an antidepressant, which did help, but I was still left with low self-esteem as a mother, and I had a lot of self-doubt, anxiety, and fears. As time went on it got more out of control, so I finally agreed to get help again. But this time I really wanted to get better and was willing to get counseling on a regular basis. Once I was willing to make lifestyle changes and learned how to think more positively and really educate myself on OCD, I was able to get off the medicine, and I actually live a happier, more positive lifestyle. I go to group meditation classes that offer great tools that I use in my daily life. I can honestly say that going through all that I went through was a blessing in disguise because I learned to love myself and life and be a better person.

Now, five years later, I am pregnant. Even the pregnancy is so much easier this time because of all the tools I learned from before. I am six months pregnant right now, and I've gotten counseling twice just as kind of a check-in. It's been nice and reassuring that I've been doing so well. I have discussed with my doctor that I will go on an antidepressant at thirty-six weeks of pregnancy as an extra precaution. For now, I just take one day at a time and know that I am as prepared as I can possibly be, and I have a great support team of my husband, my in-laws, and my mom's best friend, who actually had the same type of experience as me. They are all aware of what I went through and are willing to help me. I'm absolutely sure it will be a more positive experience this time.

Remember: Surrounding yourself with a support team and having a plan that includes therapy are keys to feeling good about yourself and your decisions.

As stated before, feeling confident and secure about the decisions you've made goes a long way toward helping you deal with people who question your judgment. However, since there aren't enough long-term studies yet on the effects of antidepressants on children whose moms took some type of psychiatric medication in pregnancy, it can be easy for doubt to creep in. Follow-up studies that we do have are reassuring, though, and practitioners who specialize in the field feel comfortable continuing to prescribe these medications to pregnant women who need them. On the positive side, some psychiatric medications are even considered "neuro-protective" (protective of the nervous system in some way) and may actually play a role in aiding brain development and preventing disorders, an area currently under study. And we know that stress hormones elevated in a depressed pregnant woman affect the baby in utero and may last for years. The point is, there is just as much information to support the possibility that an antidepressant taken in pregnancy may be a positive thing for the baby as there is to support possible danger to the baby. (In chapter 6 you can see the outcomes of the research, and the medication categories will be discussed in greater detail.) There are no guarantees with any choice, and there are possible risks with any of them. So whatever you decide, go with it and feel good about it.

But what to do when those doubts creep in? I'm a big believer in affirmations—that is, when they're done correctly. The way I define it, an affirmation is a positive statement that you intellectually know is true. Your heart may not accept it yet, but at least your rational head does. I suggest writing down a list of these statements so they'll be at your fingertips when you need them. For instance, you can write affirmations like, "We're making the best decisions for our child that we can." "We are already excellent parents, and we trust ourselves." Whenever possible, say the affirmations out loud, and say them with power in your voice. The more you say these statements like you really mean them, the more their truth will sink deep inside you and help. If you use a weak, questioning voice, the affirmations won't be as helpful.

Be happy and satisfied with whatever you choose regarding your treatment options. You are making the best decision you can with the information you have now, which is all anyone can do.

If Your Partner Doesn't Agree

So you've listened to your inner voice and know that something isn't right. You want to fix it and feel better, and you want what's best for your baby, too. However, your partner is against the idea of you taking medicine while you're pregnant. How do you proceed?

Letitia, one of my clients, was put in precisely this situation as she agonized over the decision about taking an antidepressant in her third pregnancy. She had struggled with both prenatal and postpartum depression with her first two (the second time was worse), and she swore she'd never let herself go through that again. She had wanted to take an antidepressant both times, but her family—mainly her husband, parents, and siblings—guilt-tripped and shamed her until she gave up. Letitia told me that she had allowed them to make her feel so weak that she couldn't stand her ground. "It just wasn't worth fighting them anymore," she told me. "They didn't care how bad I felt no matter how much I tried to explain it. After a few months, I just gave up trying and did my best without the medicine." Her family had drilled into her the words, "Our people are strong. Just pull it together. We don't need help like that." Those words rang loudly in her ears, but she showed her real strength by deciding to ignore

> Because culturally Letitia was taught to adhere to her husband's wishes, she was torn up inside and very confused. She really wanted her husband to accept and approve of her decision.

them this time and do what she felt was right. The hardest part for Letitia was that her husband, Amal, aligned with her family and their way of thinking. At first, he totally refused to even have a discussion about it. Because culturally Letitia was taught to adhere to her husband's wishes, she was torn up inside and very confused. She really wanted her husband to accept and approve of her decision. Since Amal was a scientist, I advised Letitia to bring Amal a few scientific papers on the subject of depression in pregnancy. These articles discussed the research that demonstrates that depression in pregnancy is biochemical and not the result of a personality weakness. The research also listed the possible risks to the developing baby if a pregnant woman goes untreated. One of the studies also outlined the risks for postpartum depression if prenatal depression isn't treated adequately. It continued on to say how children are at risk of developmental problems if the primary caretaker is depressed. Thankfully, Amal read the articles.

My next suggestion to Letitia was to invite Amal to accompany her to the psychiatrist appointment, so that Amal could ask whatever questions he might have. He agreed. What happened at that appointment was enough to sway Amal into supporting his wife's choice and to stand up for her at family gatherings. This was a monumental victory for Letitia, and she felt extremely relieved. With Letitia's permission, I had called the psychiatrist in advance to give him a heads-up about the situation, and the psychiatrist was prepared to give the couple a few extra minutes for questions or explanations. Three important things happened at that appointment. One, by coming to the doctor's office with his wife, Amal heard straight from the M.D. exactly what Letitia had already heard regarding the benefits and safety of using the medication, so he had the same information. Second, the psychiatrist was able to answer all Amal's questions in an objective way that Amal was able to accept and respect. And third, by hearing from a medical doctor (the doctor is male, which in this case was an added bonus) that Letitia would recover faster with emotional support from her husband, Amal was able to understand that he played a very important role in his family's well-being. Letitia did start taking medication the next day, and within three weeks she began to function as her previously happy self.

Most partners, I've found over the years, may have a preference to avoid medication if possible, but typically they are supportive of the woman's decision no matter which way she chooses. It's important that your partner understands how valuable his support is to you during this difficult time. Let him know that what you need to hear from him is, "Whatever you need to do in order to feel 100 percent, I'm behind you." Hopefully you already have your partner's support or are on your way to receiving it. But whether you do or don't, empower yourself. Your family

> It's important that your partner understands how valuable his support is to you during this difficult time.

needs you to be happy and whole. Only you know how you feel on the inside; you're the expert of your own experience. Therefore, no matter what, you need to give yourself full permission to make the final decision in the end, no matter what anybody else thinks. To do otherwise would be irresponsible.

If Your OB Doesn't Agree

Your OB needs to be informed if you're taking a medication, but he or she doesn't need to agree with your decision. As long as the OB accepts your decision (which is different from liking it) and doesn't make you feel uncomfortable about taking medication, then it should work out fine. If you're on a medication when you deliver, then the pediatrician should also be informed so that he or she can watch your baby for any mild side effects. Refer to chapter 2 for a more thorough discussion about how to handle it when your doctor disagrees with your choices.

What Partners and Other Close Supporters Need to Know

How to Support Her

Of course you care very much about her and want the best for both her and the baby. You might be researching various treatment options on your own and forming opinions and preferences regarding what she should do. Ideally, the two of you are in agreement about what option(s) to choose if she's depressed or suffers from anxiety. Being on the same page certainly makes the situation simpler, but it sometimes doesn't work out that way. This section offers tips to help you directly, as well as to help you support her, and therefore your relationship with her.

Your support is very important to her psychologically and emotionally. If you aren't in agreement with her thinking, it's crucial to know how to approach the topic in order to avoid hurting her feelings and damaging the relationship. What's most important now is that the two of you maintain closeness and trust. The following are two examples of common situations illustrated by two of my clients' experiences.

Athena was pregnant, quite depressed, and very conflicted when she contacted me. She was trying some natural healing methods that helped her to a point, but not enough. She reluctantly decided to go on medication. It was a hard decision for her, and she had wrestled with it for quite a while. Athena lived with her mother (she has since married), who was her closest support. Her mother, a lactation consultant, was adamantly opposed to Athena taking medication since she believed Athena would not be able to breast-feed after the baby was born. Her mother's strong words scared Athena and made her feel guilty. I explained to Athena that there were risks either way—taking the antidepressant and not taking it. When I reminded her that only she knew how badly she was feeling—her mother did not—then she was able to take her power back and trust her decision to take the medication. Her mother's fanaticism strained their relationship considerably. Athena told me she has never felt quite the same about her mother since that stressful time. She felt that her mother was invested more in the concept of breast-feeding than she was about her daughter's health. Athena's little boy is almost a year old now, and Athena and her new family are doing well (and she did breast-feed while taking the antidepressant).

Shelley and her husband, Andre, were thinking about getting pregnant. They knew she was high risk for anxiety since during her last pregnancy she became panicky for months. She hadn't taken any medication the last time around, but acupuncture and some herbs safe for pregnancy "took the edge off," she said. Andre dreaded going through that again. He urged Shelley to consider taking medication if she started feeling anxious during this pregnancy, but Shelley was determined to avoid meds. She fought his suggestion every time he brought it up. I suggested they go together to consult with a knowledgeable psychiatrist so at least they'd receive solid information about taking medication in pregnancy. After the consultation, Shelley felt better about using medication—but only as a backup if the other natural methods didn't work. The psychiatrist reminded Shelley that high anxiety in pregnancy is not good for the growing baby. Andre handled the situation with a great deal of patience. Even though he was worried—both for Shelley and for himself—he communicated to her that he supported her decision no matter what.

I introduced Shelley and Andre to a wonderful nutritional system (see chapter 8) and EFT, the Emotional Freedom Technique (see chapter 7). Using these tools, along with therapy, Shelley did great during her pregnancy. She never needed the medication. But the important point here is that the relationship between Shelley and Andre was strengthened during the process of decision making. Even though Andre had preferred that she take the medication, he always let her know he was by her side. He knew, correctly, that ultimately the choice was hers. He let her know how much he loved her and told her that whatever she felt she had to do in order to feel good, he was behind her. He actually didn't care if she took medication or not—he just wanted her to be well and happy, for everyone's sake. Once he saw how the nutrition system, EFT, and therapy were working, he was more than satisfied.

It's Up to Her

You have a right to your opinion, but ultimately the decision is hers. Unless she is clinically not capable of making rational decisions—if she's having a manic episode or in a psychotic state—support whatever she wants to do. What she needs to hear from you is, *"I love you. You deserve to feel happy. Whatever you need to do to get yourself 100 percent well, I'm behind you."* Make the phone calls for her, drive her to the consultation appointments, and attend them yourself when appropriate. Keeping this attitude isn't easy, especially when your opinion differs from hers and you feel strongly about it. But keep in mind what's most important here—namely, your relationship with her. Of course the baby's safety is important, too, and no one cares about that more than she does. Trust that she is weighing out all the pros and cons of the treatments outlined in this book and that she will make excellent decisions. What she needs is your support, which is worth more than gold.

Be Supportive

With couples or any close support people, the attitude should be that you're making the decision together as a team. If you don't want her to follow a certain path of treatment and she chooses it anyway, you still need to stay positive and supportive. Even if she wants a baby very much and you don't, if she gets pregnant the baby is still equally yours to take care of. You wouldn't say, "I never wanted a baby, so you take care of it!" Bottom line is that you're going through these experiences together as a couple, even though you have your individual feelings about it. If she feels she needs medication and you prefer she doesn't take it, ultimately she'll decide.

And whatever happens as a result of that decision, the two of you need to walk hand in hand as a team. If, for instance, she has some side effects from the medication and feels a bit dizzy, avoid pointing out to her, "See, I told you that you shouldn't take that stuff." There must never be a shred of "I told you so" in your tone of voice or your facial expression. That could be extremely detrimental to your relationship.

Her worst fear is that she'll make a decision that will hurt the baby, and then she'll feel guilty forever and you'll always blame her. Reassure her that she's making the best decision she can for the baby. She's collected the necessary information and considered all the factors. She needs to know that you won't blame her if something goes awry. The pact you need to have with yourself and with her is that no matter what, you are a team. No blaming allowed—only support and moving forward, handling whatever comes as loving partners.

Self-Esteem

One of the symptoms of depression is low self-esteem—feeling badly about yourself. When your self-esteem drops, you tend to hurl ugly put-downs toward yourself, which makes recovery even harder. It's like beating yourself up in the middle of a boxing ring. Kicking yourself when you're already down is just plain mean. You certainly wouldn't be saying those terrible things to anyone else you love, so why do it to yourself?

Here are some steps to help you change the negative self-talk to positive, as well as other tips that will help you raise your self-esteem. Even if you're not currently depressed, these tips are useful.

Trust your intuition and do what's healthy for you. Many people, including those who love you, will try to influence your decisions and tell you what's best for you and your baby. If you're doubting your ability to make your own choices now, it's extra important that you concentrate on keeping your power and not giving it away. You can certainly ask informed people for their opinions, but the bottom line is that you are the ultimate decision maker.

Practice dealing with negativity around you (if you can't avoid it altogether) and do not take it personally. Sometimes people make ignorant or insensitive comments. Depression makes it easy to internalize those comments, which hurts self-esteem. If your cousin says, "Only crazy people go to therapy—you must be whacko!" consider the source. That's a pretty uneducated statement that has nothing to do with you and everything to do with him.

Congratulate yourself for what you are doing instead of griping to yourself about what you can't do yet. You're doing the best you can, so pat yourself on the back. As you recover, your best will get better, but it's essential that you acknowledge what you're doing now in a positive way. For instance, feel good that you're able to walk to the end of the block instead of yelling at yourself about not being able to walk two blocks yet. Instead, look forward to how it will feel when you are able to walk both blocks.

Respect your personal needs. If you don't, others won't either. If it's important to you that you go to bed early, then do it—regardless of how late others in your family stay up. If taking a shower every day helps you feel good, then make sure it happens, and so on.

Speak to yourself respectfully. When you "hear" that negative voice in your head, stop. When you begin thinking something like, "Other pregnant women don't go through this—what's wrong with me?" apologize to yourself and set yourself straight. Then say something like, "Lots of women go through this. I'm not alone, and I'm taking good steps to help myself recover."

Keep your expectations realistic and set yourself up for success. Depression makes every task feel overwhelming, so even things that used to be easy now feel complicated. Don't bite off more than you can chew right now. If going to the OB for a checkup and driving to the grocery store to go food shopping feels too stressful to accomplish in one day, then don't. Choose one or the other. As you recover, you'll be able to handle more like before. Feel good about what you *are* doing.

Key Points

- *Pregnancy is a vulnerable time for women both physically and emotionally, and you may find that your sensitivities are heightened even more than usual.*

- *Try to avoid major life upheavals during pregnancy. For example, now is not the time to move, add on to your house, change jobs, or make any other big changes.*

- *You are making the best decisions for you. You don't need to share any information with anyone who you're not absolutely sure will support you.*

- *There are no guarantees with any choice, and there are possible risks with any of them. So whatever you decide, go with it and feel good about it.*

Chapter 5

PREGNANCY AND MOODS

Hormones are strange buggers. The effects of estrogen and progesterone, two of the most important reproductive hormones, are unpredictable from one woman to the next. Some women feel better than ever during part or all of their pregnancy, and others are at their very worst. You never know in advance whether you'll feel great or awful during your pregnancy—each one is like a roulette wheel. (If you feel awful, by the way, this doesn't mean anything personal about you, your baby, or your relationship with your baby either now or later. You're simply feeling a physical reaction to the chemical changes in your body.) In this chapter we will uncover the myths of pregnancy, look at body image issues that may pop up, and lay out guidelines that can help you assess whether your feelings are within the normal range. You'll read about the importance of regular mood screenings throughout your pregnancy, and you'll also see a section on different types of scary thoughts you might have during your pregnancy, what they mean (and don't mean), and what to do about them.

The Biggest Myths about Pregnancy

There are a few damaging myths about pregnancy that are still hanging around today. Before I begin, I'll explain what I mean by a myth. I'm using the term *myth* to describe a belief that there is only one way things should be, and that if you're not looking, sounding, or feeling that particular way, it means there's something deficient or inadequate about you. Of course, with any one of the myths I'm about to mention, some women do experience pregnancy this way. The problem comes when a woman expects herself to feel, look, and sound the way the "myth" describes. Then, if her experience is different from that scenario, she feels she doesn't measure up.

One of these harmful myths is the assumption that you'll be glowing and happy while you're pregnant. The images on television and in magazines of smiling women in white satin flowing gowns, looking adoringly at their burgeoning tummies, still prevail. When was the last time you saw an image of a woman in her third trimester hanging her head over the toilet with morning sickness or an anxiety-ridden woman too panicky to leave the house? Probably never. That's one of the reasons that women who aren't feeling great either physically or emotionally often feel like outsiders.

Another myth of pregnancy is that it's easy to get pregnant in the first place. The assumption that many people have is that once you decide to get pregnant, you'll get pregnant. Women frequently try to plan the month they want to conceive so the baby will be born at a convenient time in their schedule, like during summer vacation. It may or may not work out that way. That certainly isn't true for many women, especially those with infertility challenges. Along with this myth comes another: Once you're pregnant, you'll stay pregnant. Many of you reading this book, I'm sure, have experienced otherwise.

The last myth I would like to mention is the belief that pregnancy protects you from mood disorders. Just a few years ago, medical students were still taught that the high level of estrogen present during pregnancy keeps women happy. Even today, many doctors tell their patients that they won't need medication during pregnancy. Their patients who are doing well but know they're high risk are often told not to worry, since the pregnancy hormones will protect them. Those who are on medication for depression are told they can wean off before they become pregnant or stop taking the medication if they become pregnant while still on the medication. And if women are still suffering or they relapse, doctors sometimes tell them they can't take any medication since these doctors don't know the research and are worried about an unknown risk. These women are told they must suffer through their entire pregnancy, which is sad at best and dangerous for the babies and women at the worst.

What's Normal?

Over the last twenty years, many, many women have called me sometime during their pregnancy to ask if their feelings are normal. After a quick assessment, I'm able to tell them. Sometimes their feelings are normal, and sometimes not. But the point is that it's essential for the right questions to be asked. One should never assume. Often well-meaning doctors dismiss what is in fact a mood disorder as being normal. They miss the boat because they don't know what to ask or what to look for.

Andrea's Story

I am thirty-eight years old and have a beautiful four-year-old daughter and an amazing husband. We live in suburbia in a wonderful part of the country, and I am lucky enough to be able to stay home with our daughter. Eight months ago, my life seemed perfect from the outside, but I felt like something was still missing. I wanted to have another child so badly and was having difficulty getting pregnant. It had been eighteen months since we began trying, and I had had two miscarriages in a six-month period. I went through fertility testing, and the doctors could find nothing wrong with me or my husband. I couldn't understand why I couldn't get pregnant. I had been praying day after day for acceptance of the plan God had for me. Nine months after my second miscarriage, I finally accepted that it was okay if we have only one child. Our daughter is happy and healthy, and we love her. That is all that matters. But I wasn't going to stop trying to get pregnant.

I did not want to go through traditional fertility treatments such as IVF for numerous reasons. I have always been open to non-Western medicine, so I began to see an acupuncturist who specialized in fertility. It was tiring making the forty-five-minute drive each way two to three times a week for my acupuncture treatments, but at that point I would have done almost anything to have another child. Three months after beginning acupuncture I found out we *were pregnant. Words cannot describe how excited I was, but I found myself trying not to get too excited because I could still miscarry. It was April, and I was eighteen weeks and still pregnant. I was so thankful to be blessed with another child, but I was not feeling very cheerful. I was lonely, did not want to go outside, and just felt like crying all the time. I could not understand why I was feeling this way when I had so much to be happy for. In the past I had taken antidepressants, but I went off them. Like so many other people, I had placed a stigma on taking antidepressants—I thought only "crazy" people took them and that I didn't need them and should be able to handle life on my own. So I tried other ways to help me feel better, such as diet changes and changing my attitude/thought processes. However, with the help of my therapist I came to realize that there is nothing wrong with taking medication. Not only was I miserable, but I was making my husband and daughter's lives miserable. I deserve to be happy, too. So at week eighteen of my pregnancy I began taking antidepressants again. Just two weeks after beginning my medication I could feel the difference. I was laughing, enjoying the time I have with my daughter, and, most importantly, enjoying life again.*

Remember: Don't let the fear of being stigmatized prevent you from reaching out for the help you need. You deserve to be happy.

WARNING SIGNS

It's important to be able to tell if you've crossed the line and need help, so in the following pages I'll lay out some guidelines. In general, the severity of your uncomfortable feelings, their frequency, and the length of time they last are good indications of whether or not they are "normal." For instance, a mild bout of weepiness lasting fifteen minutes a day is normal, but deep sadness for a few hours every day is not. Another rule is that during a pregnancy, your mood may go up and down, but you should generally feel good about yourself. If your self-esteem is poor and you feel much more down about yourself than up, that's not normal.

For example, one of my clients, Allison, described herself to me as a "cup half full" kind of person, and she was just as quick to acknowledge her own accomplishments as she was with complimenting other people. She was positive and fun to be around. Therefore she was surprised and unnerved when she found herself slowly spiraling lower and lower, and talking down to herself frequently. At the end of her second trimester she contacted me. "I feel like Eeyore, and I used to be Tigger," she said. "I don't look forward to anything anymore, and I expect things to go wrong. I've also started being really mean to myself."

It's great that Allison recognized that this wasn't normal for her and that she reached out for help. Awareness is the first step. No changes can be made unless you know there's something that needs changing. Depression can be a little tougher to recognize if your self-esteem was on the lower side before pregnancy, unlike in Allison's situation. But if your self-talk is more negative than usual for you, or you're beating yourself up and feel rotten much of the day, call a qualified therapist. Even if you've always been hard on yourself or negative, now's a perfect time to get help so that pattern doesn't continue. You deserve to feel better. It will also be better for the next generation to have positive parents to model.

Disruptions to your sleep cycle are another warning sign. Sleep problems due to a full bladder or some heartburn may awaken you once or twice during the night. But if you have a hard time falling asleep, staying asleep, or if you wake up much too early in the morning and can't go back to sleep, this isn't normal. That is to say, if you're up and can't sleep due to sadness or worry, get help. If you're awake because of digestion problems, a full bladder, or trouble getting comfortable, this is normal for pregnancy.

> If you're up and can't sleep due to sadness or worry, get help. If you're awake because of digestion problems, a full bladder, or trouble getting comfortable, this is normal for pregnancy.

Beverly, another of my clients, experienced this. She went to her OB for a prenatal checkup and reported that she had trouble sleeping. Her OB replied, "Of course you're having trouble sleeping—you're eight months pregnant." The OB assumed that she was physically uncomfortable and that's the reason why she was having trouble. Actually, she wasn't that uncomfortable, and she was physically quite able to sleep. The problem was that the inside of her head wouldn't allow her to sleep. She was too anxious. The OB should have asked her a simple follow-up question and not just assumed that her sleep issue was normal. He should have asked, "Do you know the reason why you're having trouble sleeping?" Beverly would have told him that she was really worried about becoming a mother because she was fearful that she'd abuse the baby the same way her mother had abused her. But he never asked, and she left the office severely anxious and needing therapy. It was only after her delivery when she was in the throes of a full-blown panic disorder that her doctor finally understood that she needed help. Beverly called me five weeks into her nightmare, and now she is able to sleep and to enjoy her new life as a mom. Make sure that your doctor is "hearing" you if you think you need help. Don't allow your feelings to be dismissed if you believe something isn't right. Feeling tired is normal during pregnancy, but when you lie down and rest, you should regain your energy. However, if no amount of rest helps to restore your energy and relieve your fatigue, that's not normal. Depression causes sluggishness and tiredness that doesn't go away with rest—it zaps your energy.

> It's normal to feel some nervousness—maybe about labor, becoming a mother, or having another child. However, you should be able to experience excitement and joy. If you can't, this isn't normal.

It's normal to feel some nervousness—maybe about labor, becoming a mother, or having another child. However, you should be able to experience excitement and joy. If you can't, this isn't normal. When your anxiety is high, it's very difficult to feel any happiness. You're too busy worrying, and it takes over your head.

Typically in pregnancy, appetite increases. If you find that your appetite actually decreases, or you lose your appetite completely, that's not normal. If this happens to you, it's important to make yourself eat (healthfully). Your body still needs food even if you're not feeling hungry. Refer to chapter 8 for a discussion on a nutrition system that will feed your brain chemistry and help to keep your moods stable.

SCARY THOUGHTS

Many pregnant women occasionally have thoughts that disturb them. These thoughts take various forms, and a thought that bothers one woman may not bother the next. For instance, the thought "I regret getting pregnant—I don't think I want to be a mother" is quite normal when it occurs once in a while. One minute you may be excited about the baby, and the next minute you may realize how much your life is going to change and want to turn back the clock to a time before you got pregnant. That type of thought scares some women and only mildly annoys other women. If any particular thought you're having scares you, ask a professional (a therapist would be my first choice) if the thought is normal. Maybe all you need is reassurance to be able to stop worrying about it. The frequency, severity, and duration of the thoughts will let you know if you're within normal range or if you need some intervention. A brief period of mild worry once or twice a week is normal; a few hours of full-fledged anxiety daily is not. The rule of thumb is, if the thoughts are getting in the way of you enjoying your life, get help.

A tough but important topic to cover is thoughts of harming yourself. These thoughts fall into two basic groups: One type of thought isn't dangerous (at least not yet), and the other one is. For example, you may think of running away or escaping from your life in some way, which is what I call an "escapist fantasy." It's not necessarily a dangerous thought. You don't actually want to die; you just don't want to be in pain anymore. You don't want to live like this, and you want to leave all your problems somewhere else and run. I remember fantasizing about getting on a bus in California, where I live, and riding it all the way to the other side of the country. When I'd think these thoughts, I'd feel an immediate relief. Even though these thoughts aren't necessarily dangerous, you still should get some professional help if you have them since you're probably depleted and burned out physically and emotionally. You need a plan to recharge yourself.

Another type of escapist fantasy can mean trouble, however. This includes thoughts like, "If a bus hit me or I just didn't wake up tomorrow morning, that would be okay." The thought, even though it comes from a very sad place, can feel like a relief. You wouldn't actually take the steps to hurt yourself, but you feel like if you were to disappear, it would be fine. Those thoughts can spiral down into serious suicidal thoughts if you don't get help. You're flirting with danger here, so tell a health care provider about these feelings right away.

If a person is actively suicidal, that means she is capable, willing, and even planning to actually take the physical steps to kill herself. These are not escapist fantasies anymore— these are suicidal thoughts. These are the most serious, and a woman in this situation needs professional help yesterday. She is in imminent danger and shouldn't be left alone for a minute until she's more stable.

Stay Positive

Surrounding yourself with a positive environment is always healthy, but it's especially important when you're dealing with depression or are experiencing a vulnerable period in your life. It will strengthen the solid foundation you need to keep yourself mentally and emotionally well. "Environment" consists of all that surrounds you: house, sounds, colors, clothes, people—everything.

Abby contacted me in her seventh month of pregnancy. She was thinking about taking an antidepressant but wanted to know if there were alternatives to help her get through the pregnancy. As part of her initial assessment, I asked Abby if she watches TV or listens to the radio. She told me that she doesn't actually watch very much TV or listen to much of what the radio was broadcasting, but one or the other of these boxes was on as background noise almost constantly, just to keep her company. She told me that silence was scary to her because she felt alone, and also the negative thoughts in her head got too "loud." She used the TV and radio as company and as a distraction. When I asked her what stations she had on, it turned out that they were the channels and frequencies that broadcast the most abysmal, sensationalistic, fear-producing "information." The negativity filling her house and her mind, as her attention tuned in and out of what the shows were communicating, was bringing her down. She hadn't realized it consciously until I gave her an assignment: I asked her to put on uplifting, *fun music and motivational tapes instead of the usual programs she was used to. She could also rent funny movies instead of TV. Within one week (it was technically five days), the difference in her mood was dramatic. She was hopeful, laughing again, and having fun with her older children. She left the room when her husband watched the news (often the worst type of negativity) and put on her headphones with great music. This single change may not be the only one needed for everyone to return to normal, but my point is, don't underestimate how powerful words and messages are. Even if you're not completely "tuned in," they are still affecting you in a huge way!*

Depression and anxiety can make you more sensitive in general. With the added hormonal fluctuations, these sensitivities can be even more heightened. If you're easily bothered by rough fabrics, for example, indulge yourself by dressing in soft clothing. This might sound silly, but it can make a big difference in your stress and irritability level by the end of the day.

If normal sounds around you have started to annoy you, wear headphones or earplugs (when safe to do so, of course) to tone it down a few notches. This works great with a newborn, too, by the way. You'll be able to hear your baby when she really needs you, but the shrill cries won't make your skin crawl and your stomach tie up in knots.

Getting light (especially sunlight) during the day can make a big difference in your mood. You

*don't have to spend hours outside—just a few min-
utes of sunlight every day can give you a boost. If
it's raining or gray and gloomy, turn on some extra
lights in your room and watch what happens to
your happiness level. (If you're more anxious than
depressed, bright light can be overstimulating, so
adjust it accordingly.)*

*Be careful what you're reading as well. Avoid
the pregnancy manuals that are so purist that they
scare you into thinking that one piece of chocolate
during your pregnancy will damage your baby-to-
be. (There are other things that you should absolutely and completely avoid, but chocolate isn't one
of them.) I recommend that you steer clear of guilt-
tripping magazines that communicate, "if you
don't sign your child up for preschool before she's
born, she'll never get in!" And, above all, no newspapers. This is almost as bad as watching the news
on TV. There is rarely anything positive in newspapers since negativity and fear are what drive sales.
Instead, read pleasurable books and magazines
that give you a minivacation from your mind and
take you away to another place. Read fun material
that makes you laugh, motivational books, or fluffy
novels.*

*Energy is "catching," so choose your company
wisely. Avoid the naysayers, gossips, and critics—
their energy is like poison. Invite upbeat and positive relatives and friends to your home and out
to lunch, and don't accept invitations or initiate
contact with negative people. I know this can be a*

bit more complicated when it involves close family members, so just do your best. If you live with someone negative, make it your own assignment to model positive talk, and that means no complaining whatsoever.

Complaining is toxic. By all means, if there's something you don't like in your life, then take charge and try to fix it, or change your perspective about it so you can be more positive. Complaining makes you a victim—as if you have no power to change a situation or your attitude about it. Don't allow yourself to do that. Certainly you should show compassion for yourself, as you would anyone else you love, but that's not complaining—that's allowing your feelings and accepting them. It's what you do next that makes the difference. Continuing to spin in circles of complaints doesn't get you anywhere but miserable.

OBSESSIVE-COMPULSIVE DISORDER

One of the mood disorders that can happen in pregnancy is obsessive-compulsive disorder (OCD). This anxiety disorder causes intense recurrent, unwanted thoughts (obsessions) or rituals (compulsions), which people suffering from it feel they cannot control. Rituals such as hand washing, counting, checking, or cleaning are often performed in hope of preventing obsessive thoughts or making them go away. There are scary thoughts often associated with OCD in pregnancy and postpartum, and these thoughts can be disabling, depending on the severity of the episode. Although OCD is not always accompanied by these thoughts, they happen frequently enough and are scary enough to warrant this section. It's important for you to know what's happening if you recognize yourself in the following scenario.

Kristin loved knowing she was pregnant. She and her husband, Stephen, started making plans for their baby when she was still in her first trimester. When she was about seven weeks pregnant, however, Kristin started having disturbing thoughts of her baby dying. As if that weren't bad enough, some of these thoughts were about Kristin herself making her baby die. The worst thought she had was about sticking a kitchen knife into her abdomen. "I was so terrified. I thought I must be this monster mother. Why else would I be having these horrible thoughts?" Kristin had OCD, but she had never been diagnosed. After we began working together, Kristin realized that some of the behaviors and thoughts she had always had were actually related to OCD. She had always had a great attention to detail, she was a perfectionist who needed to keep her home spotless, and she would often anticipate danger in any situation, no matter how harmless. Before her pregnancy, the OCD was mildly annoying, and every month before her period she would get worse. But the symptoms never felt like they did now when she was pregnant. The thoughts of harming her baby became so debilitating that she was barely able to go to work. She was scared, guilt-ridden, and ashamed. It wasn't easy for Kristin to acknowledge her thoughts to me since she was afraid I'd call Child Protective Services. I had a feeling she was suffering from OCD even before she described what these thoughts were, and I assured her that she could trust me. I told her that I needed to know what was happening in her head so that I could give her the kind of help she needed. Along with dietary changes, sleep suggestions, and a few alterations in her schedule, I also suggested she speak with a psychiatrist about taking an antidepressant. She was reluctant (being a perfectionist), but she said anything would be better than feeling like this. Within one week after starting an SSRI ("selective serotonin reuptake inhibitor," a newer class of antidepressant drugs), the scary thoughts began to subside. She stayed on the medicine until a few months after she delivered. When the thoughts started again during her second pregnancy, she immediately went back on the same antidepressant, and she was able to avoid months of suffering.

> If a woman doesn't receive help for obsessive thoughts, there is a risk she may harm herself since she's typically very depressed and ashamed about having these thoughts.

If a woman doesn't receive help for obsessive thoughts, there is a risk she may harm herself since she's typically very depressed and ashamed about having these thoughts. The thoughts are in part due to lowered levels of the brain chemical serotonin. The woman is so afraid that harm will come to her baby that she obsesses about the most horrible fear she has: that she is the one who may bring harm to her baby. The truth is, mothers who suffer from these thoughts are actually the most protective mothers on the planet.

The scary thoughts that often accompany OCD in pregnancy or postpartum do not put the baby at risk. They are extremely frightening to the mother, but the baby is not in danger. They are only thoughts—the moms don't act on the thoughts. These women don't trust that their babies are safe until they understand it's OCD, and even then, they need a lot of reassurance that they're not psychotic. Her partner or another adult living with her will notice that she dreads being alone with the baby, and she'll become very anxious when that's about to occur. Often she'll show extreme anxiety about the baby's health and check his breathing, fix the blanket repeatedly so it doesn't cover his face, and so on. Pregnant women with psychosis, a completely different and unrelated disorder, can absolutely cause harm to the baby. Note: During her evaluation with a competent professional who understands the huge difference between OCD and psychosis, she should be screened to make sure there is no psychosis present. Although probably very rare, it's possible for these disorders to be present at the same time.

PSYCHOSIS

It is very uncommon for psychosis to arise for the first time in pregnancy. A woman who has a past history of a psychotic illness (like schizophrenia, for instance), however, may need to take antipsychotic medication during pregnancy. If she has a psychotic episode, she may not even know there's anything wrong with her. It is extremely dangerous since the woman is not in our reality. At any moment she may become delusional, thinking that she needs to kill the baby, and follow through. This woman will also be hallucinating, often hearing voices that tell her to harm her baby, herself, or both. Obviously, if she's pregnant, any attempt to harm herself would be gravely dangerous for her baby. This mom should be immediately driven to the hospital for in-patient care. If hospitalization isn't possible for some reason, then a trusted adult support person needs to be with her at all times—including in the bathroom—until she's stable. Signs of psychosis include floating in and out of a delusional state, hearing voices, paranoia, visual hallucinations, and making strange statements.

SCREENING

A staff member in your OB's office (not necessarily the doctor) should screen you for depression and anxiety every trimester. This should happen regardless of whether you've ever been clinically depressed or anxious before. If you have experienced these or any other mood disorder in the past, you're very high risk. But whether or not you have a past history of a mood disorder, it's not enough to be checked once in the pregnancy. For instance, you may have felt fine earlier the pregnancy but developed depression a few weeks later. If you aren't being regularly screened, ask why not and make sure you are. Many OB practices are already on board with this procedure and are making it a standard protocol. That's the way it should be. There are various simple screening tools used in pregnancy that take just a few minutes, like the Edinburgh Postnatal Depression Scale or the Postpartum Depression Predictors Inventory. If a formal screening instrument isn't being used, at least the staff member can ask you a few simple informal questions to assess how you're doing emotionally.

This excerpt, from *Beyond the Blues: A Guide to Understanding and Treating Prenatal and Postpartum Depression* (Bennett, Indman 2006), includes questions that you can ask yourself before you get pregnant to assess your risk, and also while you're pregnant. This informal screening tool was created so practitioners would have something easy to refer to when women are in their offices. The most important questions are listed first, followed by a bit of explanation for the practitioner. The questions that come later are also helpful, but sometimes practitioners may not have time to ask them. *Perinatal* refers to something that occurs during pregnancy and/or postpartum, and a "perinatal psychotherapist" is a therapist who specializes in the treatment of perinatal mood disorders.

- ***Have you ever had depression, panic, extreme anxiety, OCD, bipolar disorder, psychosis, or an eating disorder?*** *Women with a personal history of mood disorders need to be educated about their high risk for a perinatal mood disorder. They should be referred to a perinatal psychotherapist to help them develop a plan of action to minimize their risk. Those women with a history of bipolar disorder or psychosis should also be referred to a psychiatrist for a medication evaluation and observation during pregnancy and postpartum.*

- ***Are you taking any medications (prescription or nonprescription) or herbs on a regular basis?*** *Women who are self-treating for insomnia, anxiety, sadness, or other symptoms that may indicate a mood disorder, should be evaluated by a perinatal psychotherapist.*

- ***Have you had a previous postpartum mood disorder?*** *Women answering yes to this question are at extremely high risk for another perinatal mood disorder. They should be referred to a perinatal psychotherapist in order to develop a plan of action to prevent or at least minimize another occurrence.*

- **Have you ever taken any psychotropic medications?** *If yes, educate them about their risk of developing a perinatal mood disorder. Observe them carefully during pregnancy and postpartum.*
- **Have you ever had severe premenstrual mood changes (PMS or PMDD)?** *Women whose moods are affected by hormone changes are clearly at high risk during pregnancy and postpartum since there are dramatic hormonal shifts. Educate them about their risk, and observe them carefully during pregnancy and postpartum.*
- **Do you have any family history of mental illness?** *If yes, educate them about their risk, and observe them during pregnancy and postpartum.*
- **Do you have any personal or family history of substance abuse?**
- **Do you smoke?**
- **If pregnant, how have you been feeling physically and emotionally?**
- **Do you feel you have adequate emotional and physical support?**
- **Have you had a birth-related trauma (or other traumatic incident such as rape or sexual abuse)?**
- **Are you experiencing any major life stressors (for example, moving, job change, deaths, financial problems)?**
- **Have there been any health problems for you or the fetus?**
- **Do you have a personal or family history of thyroid disorder?**

If you've been clinically depressed or anxious in the past, it's normal (though not pleasant) to be very concerned if you feel a twinge of the old feelings. "It's the depression/anxiety returning!" you may worry. Instead of jumping to the worst conclusion, try to stay grounded in the here and now, present time. For example, it's normal to be more emotional in pregnancy, as long as it's not taking over your day and is within normal limits, as discussed above. Remember that the severity, frequency, and the duration of your feelings will be the key in determining whether or not you need intervention. You can try to calm yourself down by saying, "this is only a twinge—it doesn't mean I'm getting depressed, and it may be gone in a second."

> The severity, frequency, and the duration of your feelings will be the key in determining whether or not you need intervention.

If you're not sure that what you're experiencing is normal, get checked by a professional who has the knowledge and who also will be honest with you. Get these reality checks from a doctor, therapist, or someone else who has the expertise and can assess you and evaluate what's going on objectively—not someone who will automatically say "that's normal" because she doesn't know any better or because she's attempting to make you relax no matter what the truth of the matter is. What you're feeling may not be normal, and the lack of information will not help you. As with any other important issue, it's not the education—but the lack of education—that can harm you.

Avoiding Added Stress

During pregnancy and postpartum you are at your most vulnerable for developing a mood disorder. More stress can heighten that vulnerability even further. It is important to note that your body cannot tell the difference between good stress and bad stress: The adrenaline that shoots through your system when you're busily trying to pack and organize your house for a move may be the same as when a mugger is chasing you down the street. Consciously you're aware that the first scenario is leading to something good, as opposed to the latter negative situation, but chemically both situations can push your vulnerability over the edge into an anxious or depressed state.

Although moving to a larger house may seem like a good idea, doing so during pregnancy or shortly after the baby comes home is most definitely not the time! Over the years, countless pregnant and postpartum women have contacted me, stressed to the max, having just moved. Even though you may be excited about being able to spread out in a larger dwelling, please move either before you become pregnant or wait about six months after the baby comes, until your life—and brain chemistry—settle down a bit. Adding onto your home can be just as stressful. The job is never completed when you expect it to be (and you may deliver early), and it's chaotic, dirty, noisy, and invasive during the construction. This is also not the appropriate time for you or your husband to start a new job. Often a husband is feeling the pressure to provide financially for his growing family, and that's what prompts him to go looking for a job that pays more. But usually that job also requires him to travel more and be away from you and the children. This never pays off for the family's emotional health, so if possible, don't let this happen. His presence and support is worth more than the extra bucks.

Stress, Inflammation, and Depression

Stress causes inflammation in the immune system, and inflammation causes depression in a number of ways, including the decrease of serotonin, one of the most important brain chemicals controlling mood. Inflammation levels tend to rise at the end of pregnancy, during the last trimester, and add to that all the common stresses associated with being a new mother—including labor and delivery, sleep deprivation, hormone shifts, role changes, and pain—and you have a collision course for increased inflammation. Interestingly, SSRI antidepressants lower inflammation, in addition to the other ways in which they help alleviate depression, and Cognitive Behavioral Therapy (CBT) and Interpersonal Therapy (IPT) lower inflammation as well. Negative emotions like resentment, frustration, and anger cause inflammation (thus causing depression), and one theory about the effectiveness of talk therapy is that it lowers inflammation in the body as it helps the person to release negative emotions.

Body Image

Cultural views on beauty standards regarding weight can be a whole book in and of itself. Women in various countries and cultures look upon American women and their poor body image during pregnancy in disbelief, since they are raised feeling that pregnancy is when a woman's body is the most voluptuous and sexy. In other countries, women who are nine months pregnant are photographed wearing thong bikinis for fashion magazines, whereas American women often wear "I'm not fat, I'm pregnant" T-shirts to make sure they won't be judged.

In addition, how much weight you're supposed to gain in pregnancy is pretty confusing, and it varies depending upon whom you ask. Trust your doctor, since the answer depends on your individual situation. How you may feel about your body during pregnancy is based on many factors—previous beliefs and "programming" about beauty and being pregnant, for example. You may have a tough time with weight gain during pregnancy, no matter how much or how little weight you're told to put on. Even though you know rationally that it's a necessity to gain weight for the health of the baby, it may go against what you've always tried hard to do—not gain weight.

On the other hand, you may feel liberated because now you have full permission to eat all those "forbidden" foods. You may feel relieved that the pressure is off, and you can relax about the number of calories or amount of fat you're consuming. You may feel sexier than ever, appreciating your full breasts and whole body more than you ever did previously.

If you have a history of an eating disorder, you're high risk for a recurrence during pregnancy. If you are trying not to eat or you're binging and purging in order to stay thin, for your sake and your baby's sake, get help immediately. It's easy to start denying or rationalizing these behaviors, so the faster you receive proper professional guidance, the better off your whole family will be. You are also at high risk for a mood disorder in pregnancy or postpartum (or both). If you've experienced depression, you know that low self-esteem (along with self-criticism), worry, and increased vulnerability go along with it. Depression can alter appetite dramatically in either direction, so your weight gain may not be appropriate—too much or too little weight gain may be the result. Body image issues on top of depression or even caused by the depression can be extra difficult during pregnancy. This is another example of when therapy can be very helpful. Sometimes just having a time and place to talk through these feelings is enough to put your mind at ease.

Key Points

- *Contrary to popular belief, pregnancy does not protect you from mood disorders.*

- *The severity of your uncomfortable feelings, their frequency, and the length of time they last are good measures of whether or not they are "normal."*

- *Surrounding yourself with a positive environment will strengthen the solid foundation you need to keep yourself mentally and emotionally well.*

- *Get screened for depression and anxiety every trimester.*

Chapter 6

ANTIDEPRESSANTS AND OTHER MEDICINES FOR MOOD DISORDERS

This chapter discusses the various medication categories outlined by the Federal Drug Administration (FDA),
what they mean (and what they don't mean), and what's
important to know as you make your medication decisions. I'll also give you some tips regarding the media
scares that have hit the public regarding the safety of
medication in pregnancy and help you understand what
to pay attention to and what to ignore.

As you read through the section that addresses the
possible risks of taking medications during pregnancy,
please keep in mind that there are also risks associated
with not taking the medication. First, researchers know
that the internal environment for the growing baby is
impacted when the pregnant mother is depressed or
anxious. (Exactly how the baby is affected is under study
now, but the theory is that there are chemical and hormonal changes that occur when the pregnant mother is
depressed or anxious that affect the baby's development

negatively.) Second, it's hard to take care of yourself properly when you're feeling depressed or anxious, and that's not healthy for anyone concerned, particularly when you are pregnant. Also remember that the general population has a 3 to 5 percent risk of having a child with a birth defect, whether or not the mother is taking a psychiatric medication. As my trusted psychiatrist friend and copresenter Dr. Phyllis Cedars says, "Pregnancy is a risky business!" Even when women do everything they can to give their babies every possible health advantage during pregnancy, sometimes things still go wrong, and it is nobody's fault. It is important to know that sad medical outcomes occur, and if they happen to you, you and your family need to understand you are not alone, and you are not to blame.

Medication Is Never Enough

The human body is magnificent. When it's fed properly and taken care of well in all respects—physically, emotionally, spiritually, and psychologically—it usually does a wonderful job in healing itself and remaining well. I don't believe that medication should necessarily be the first or only method tried when treating mood disorders. In the United States, one out of every four adult women is prescribed an antidepressant at some point in her life. That's a staggering 25 percent. Women are most vulnerable to mood disorders during the reproductive years, so it makes sense that many pregnant women are prescribed psychiatric medication.

The purpose of psychiatric medications is not to change you. You already feel "changed" and not yourself when you are suffering from a mood disorder. Their purpose is to help you feel more like "you," so that you can live the life you would otherwise lead without being impacted by the mood or anxiety disorder. The field of neuroscience has rapidly advanced over the past few decades, and researchers have recently identified actual areas in the brain that function differently when individuals are depressed and been able to see how successful treatment restores brain function. Mood and anxiety disorders, with the neurochemical and hormonal changes associated with them, are medical conditions, and there is no shame in receiving treatment for them. Depending on your particular situation, it's entirely possible that you won't be on the medication long-term. Medication can help you out of crisis as you get your life back on track and the other pieces of your treatment plan are improved. However, even if it seems unlikely that you'll need medication at all, you should know what's out there so you'll have a working knowledge in case medication becomes a necessity.

In this chapter I have outlined the main types of psychiatric medications. Please know that *all* medications have possible side effects and risks. There are certainly risks of untreated mood disorders as well, so treatment is important—it's a matter of what method(s) of treatment will be used. Ideally, medication should be prescribed as part of a comprehensive treatment plan that includes psychotherapy. If therapy is not an option, then the plan should include other ways to bolster support.

Psychiatric medications are probably overprescribed—but they're sometimes underprescribed. Some women who would greatly benefit from medication never receive the screening, diagnosis, and treatment that they need, and many individuals suffer for decades before getting treatment (if they ever get it at all). Stigma, access to health care, and fears about medication risk sometimes limit whether a woman receives or accepts treatment with medication.

Mood and anxiety disorders, with the neurochemical and hormonal changes associated with them, are medical conditions, and there is no shame in receiving treatment for them.

On the other hand, many physicians have too little time per patient, too little knowledge about psychiatric disorders, and limited understanding of non-medication treatments. Our fragmented health care system and providers with various perspectives and training often results in far less teamwork than is needed between physicians and mental health practitioners. This often results in the overprescribing of medication.

To complicate this issue further, there has been a rising awareness about the relationships between physicians and the pharmaceutical industry. The medical profession has come under increased scrutiny from within and from the outside, questioning how gifts from the drug companies can influence doctors' prescription habits. In fact, medical schools are now questioning even the smallest gifts to students, such as pens and lunches. Also, there are sometimes complicated relationships between doctors and these companies in regard to educational programs and research. Ideally, companies and researchers would work together to find treatment options that are safe and effective for women. Marketing in the health care industry should have clear boundaries and accountability, so when your doctor is writing prescriptions for you, you can trust fully that only your best interests are in mind.

Again, a prescription for psychiatric medication should be only part of a treatment plan—the complete answer to what you need is not found in a bottle. It is only part of the picture. All the antidepressants in the world won't replace finding long-lasting solutions to your problems, changing your mindset, increasing your support, and a implementing a healthy lifestyle. Therapy can help improve your quality of life on many levels, including your coping skills, your relationships, and gaining greater clarity on what you want in life. Exercise and nutrition are important for everyone and are necessary for optimal health and recovery from almost every medical condition, including mood and anxiety disorders. Ironically, it's taken many years for medical professionals to finally recognize that mood disorders in pregnancy and postpartum are real, clinical, biochemical disorders. Now, at least, doctors are usually willing to prescribe, and that's a good thing when it's really necessary.

Many women suffer from chronic or recurrent mood disorders, and some women will need to remain on medication for the long term. If you have experienced multiple serious episodes of depression and need your medication to stay well, please remember that this is fine. In fact, sticking closely to a regimen that works for you is a gift to yourself and your family. Suffering from depression robs you and your family of joyful and fulfilling life experiences that can never be replaced.

Not every woman with depression will need medication, or at least not for long. But if you do, consider it a valid part of your plan for wellness and allow yourself to benefit from that option without guilt or shame.

I'm grateful that these medications have been developed, so that when a woman needs them to function, they're there. Especially when a woman is in crisis, such as with severe and frequent panic attacks, it's good that she can have in her hands a pill that can quell her anxiety within ten minutes. If she's willing and able to learn psychotherapeutic techniques, work on her nutrition, change the thoughts she dwells on, and add other modalities mentioned in chapter 7, she may be able to wean off her medication entirely or at least cut down on the dosage. However, until she feels more functional, more herself, and has the ability to use more natural healing methods to take care of the root of her health issues, it's wonderful that she has medication at her disposal that can help her immediately.

If You're On a Medication or Thinking about It

If you've reviewed all your choices and considered the factors involved in making a decision by using this book and consulting with your team of professionals, and you've decided to go on (or stay on) a particular medication, feel good about it. It takes a lot of energy to weigh everything out. You're making the best decision you feel is right for you and your growing family, and that's very important. And you're working with a doctor whose expertise you can trust. If you're doing well now and you're just exploring your options for treatment should you need it later on, applaud yourself. If you take a thorough look at all that's offered, you'll be in a much more informed position when and if you need to choose some method(s) of treatment. Meanwhile, take a look at the Prevention of Postpartum Mood Disorders section in chapter 9.

What Do the Drug Classifications Really Mean?

Before I outline the drug classifications, I want to help you understand the meaning (or lack thereof) of what you'll be seeing. Otherwise, it's easy to become confused or concerned when there's no need to be. The FDA drug classifications rank medications in categories A, B, C, D, and X (with A being the least risky and X being the most risky), and these classifications are found in the PDR. They are of limited value according to most experts who devote their professional careers to this field.

The American College of Obstetricians and Gynecologists (ACOG) bulletin (Vol. 7, No. 4/April 2008) comments that the FDA pregnancy categories have many shortcomings. Most psychiatrists who specialize in treating pregnant women know the limitations of this rating system. For instance, no psychotropic drug is category A; most are C or D—without meaningful distinctions between the categories. They are usually not based on adequate human data (mainly the data is from animals), and they fail to include the risks of untreated mood disorders in pregnancy for the mother and baby. They are often out of date. The only psychiatric medication that currently has a B rating is clozapine, based on almost no human data. This is ironic, because while it is a powerful and often profoundly effective antipsychotic medication, it has very serious side effects, far beyond those of antidepressants. This particular medication would almost never be prescribed to a pregnant woman. In fact, the risk of decreased white blood cells (necessary for the body's immune system) is so high with clozapine that users of this medication need to have regular blood monitoring every one to two weeks. Yet it's in a "safer" category than antidepressants, which are prescribed on a regular basis and have few to no problems associated with them.

The clearest example of the need to drop the FDA system was when bupropion (Wellbutrin), which had been a category B medication, was moved to category C in 2006. The use of bupropion in pregnant patients has limited data and very small animal samples to support its safety (a category is often determined from animal and not human data), so this move made sense in that context. At the same time, however, SSRIs such as fluoxetine (Prozac) and citalopram (Celexa) are category C even though more than two thousand women who provided data took them in the first trimester and there is evidence of their safety. SSRIs commonly prescribed in pregnancy have a large database of information from women, which is a lot more reliable than animal data. The category changes are very slow, way behind what experienced doctors already know, adding to the belief that this system is less than useful. Although it is challenging, the only way for professionals to help women decide what is in their best interest regarding medication in pregnancy is to stay up-to-date on an evolving area of research—requiring a level of dedication and expertise that not all medical doctors will have. That is why it is so important to see someone who has the necessary expertise to treat pregnant women.

When a drug in the United States is being developed for pregnant women, it requires extensive testing before it goes on the market. Animal studies are used to help in this research in order to evaluate the effects of the drug on the reproductive system. Plus, information is gathered about the effects of the drug on babies born from women who used the drug in pregnancy. These methods don't clearly reveal the appropriate dosage considered safe in pregnancy, so it's assumed to be the typical adult dosage given when not pregnant. Hopefully in the future there will be more advice and detailed information provided right on the drug label regarding the possible risks of taking the drug while pregnant.

Before we get to the FDA category system, it's important that you know how to interpret it. Excellent doctors warn their patients not to take the categories too literally. Each decision about whether to take a medication should be based much more on an individual, case-by-case basis rather than on the category to which the medication is assigned. If, after a thorough assessment by your doctor and specialized therapist, you decide that medication would be a good choice for you, then go with it.

One of the most important reasons for working with a doctor who has great clinical expertise in this area is because these doctors treat "outside of the box" all the time. The most excellent doctors I know are using certain psychiatric medications, combinations of medications, and dosages in ways that aren't yet laid out by the FDA. You want a doctor who can tailor a regimen that works specifically for you as an individual, as opposed to the cookie-cutter way right out of the book—the *Physician's Desk Reference* (PDR).

The good news is that the FDA is in the process of completely redoing their labeling system for medications used in pregnancy. However, this overhaul will take years, and, in the meantime, many physicians are still not up to speed with the limitations of the PDR when referring to it for medications in pregnancy.

Although I obviously believe you should be an informed consumer, some information may not be helpful. Specifically, you may want to think twice before looking at the drug category assigned to your medication. For the same reasons I also advise my clients—especially those dealing with anxiety and obsessiveness—not to read the inserts that the pharmacist places in the bag with their medication. This is where trust in your prescribing doctor comes in. She is helping to evaluate what is safest for you and your baby. Certainly you should ask questions if you have them; just know that the answers can be quite confusing. With all that said, I'll outline the categories here so you'll be informed. Just take the information with a grain of salt. As a matter of fact, feel free to skip the chart entirely. If you've already examined all your options and decided that medication should be part of your treatment plan, you may be in a better position to read ahead.

FDA Categories for Medication in Pregnancy

CATEGORY A

Adequate and well-controlled studies with pregnant women have not shown there's a risk to the fetus in the first trimester of pregnancy, and there's no evidence of risk in later trimesters either.

CATEGORY B

Animal studies have revealed no evidence of harm to the fetus, but there are no adequate and well-controlled studies with pregnant women. This category can also mean that animal studies have shown a negative effect; however, adequate and well-controlled studies in pregnant women have not shown a risk to the fetus in any trimester.

CATEGORY C

Animal studies have shown a negative effect on the fetus, and there are no adequate and well-controlled studies in pregnant women. But the possible benefits may warrant the use of the drug in pregnant women despite potential risks. This category can also mean that no animal studies have been conducted and there are no adequate and well-controlled studies in pregnant women.

CATEGORY D

There is evidence in studies with pregnant women that there is a risk to the fetus. But, it may be worth the benefit to the pregnant woman to use the drug in spite of a potential risk (if she's seriously ill and nothing else may work, for instance).

CATEGORY X

Studies in animals or pregnant women have demonstrated fetal abnormalities and risks. This category means that the risk of using the drug will not outweigh the benefit—the drug should not be used by pregnant women.

Many studies have shown that the older tricyclic antidepressants and fluoxetine (Prozac) are safe in pregnancy. One excellent study found that there are no differences in the IQ, language, and temperament of children between the ages of fifteen and seventy-one months who were born to mothers who took these medications in pregnancy, as compared to the children born of nondepressed women who did not take medications in pregnancy. However, IQ and language development were negatively affected in the groups of children with depressed mothers. IQ and language development were the same for breast-fed and formula-fed children.

Research Methods

Researchers figure out what kinds of treatments work through a process of trial and error. There are three main avenues for these trials: clinical trials, case studies, and epidemiological studies.

A clinical trial is a research study that requires a design and stringent guidelines about what patients are chosen to participate and how they're chosen. An open trial requires that both the researchers and the participants know what treatment is being tested. In a double-blind trial, neither the researchers nor the patients know which treatment the participants are receiving.

Before a psychiatric medication can be sold in the United States, it needs to have several clinical trials conducted demonstrating that the medication is more effective than a placebo (such as a sugar pill or some other substance that doesn't provide benefit) for depression or another mood disorder.

A case study is an analysis of the consequences of treatment for one patient or a group of patients. Case studies are useful for uncovering areas that deserve further research. For instance, if a small group of patients are all using the same treatment and the patients respond in a similarly positive fashion, that might indicate that this treatment warrants further study. The treatment won't be "proven" until the results of large groups of participants in more studies demonstrate the same positive effect from the treatment.

Scientists use epidemiological studies in a number of ways. For example, these studies are useful if researchers are examining the risk factors of a specific disease, or if they're looking at a disease's rate of occurrence. Epidemiological studies help to foster ideas regarding how certain problems are caused and what might facilitate their treatment. This type of study does not prove cause and effect regarding cures for certain diseases, but it does indicate how factors may be related.

Specific Types of Psychiatric Medication

ANTIDEPRESSANTS

There are two main categories (although there are more) of antidepressants that are prescribed to pregnant and breast-feeding women: tricyclics (TCAs) and selective serotonin reuptake inhibitors (SSRIs). TCAs have been around since the 1950s and have more side effects than SSRIs, which are a newer type of antidepressant. Although TCAs are still prescribed frequently in pregnancy for pain, they are no longer prescribed often for depression. Assumed to work by increasing the brain's supply of norepineprine and serotonin, two brain chemicals (neurotransmitters) that affect mood, these medications are usually prescribed for women who don't respond well to the newer antidepressants.

The second category, SSRIs, boost the brain's level of serotonin, a neurotransmitter that is very important in regulating mood. This group of antidepressants has become increasingly popular ever since the original SSRI, Prozac, entered the scene in the late 1980s. Fluoxetine (Prozac), sertraline (Zoloft), paroxetine (Paxil), citalopram (Celexa), escitalopram (Lexapro), and fluvoxamine (Luvox) are among the most commonly prescribed SSRIs. Related antidepressants include duloxetine (Cymbalta), nefazodone (Serzone), and venlafaxine (Effexor). Bupropion (Wellbutrin) is also used during pregnancy, but it doesn't affect serotonin—it may affect dopamine and norepinephrine, but it's still unclear. Interestingly, bupropion is approved for smoking cessation, marketed for this use under the brand name Zyban, but is the very same drug as Wellbutrin. Obviously, smoking is known to be harmful to your baby (and to you), so if you are a smoker, that is something to consider when selecting an antidepressant. However, if you have struggled with bulimia, you should not take bupropion (because of increased risk of seizures).

While an SSRI is usually the first type of antidepressant prescribed to a pregnant woman, some (but not all) studies suggest that there may be an increased risk of fetal heart defects with paroxetine (Paxil) when used in the first trimester, so many doctors avoid prescribing it during pregnancy. Some antidepressants are well known for uncomfortable withdrawal symptoms upon cessation, including gastrointestinal and flulike symptoms, dizziness, and rebound anxiety (temporary return of the anxiety). Paroxetine and venlafaxine (Effexor) have been reported to have substantial risks of withdrawal responses with missed doses, although theoretically this could happen with most medications. Therefore, if you decide to stop your medication, do so with the knowledge and help of your doctor. Under most circumstances, tapering down slowly will help you avoid withdrawal symptoms and also help you and your doctor notice if you are becoming more depressed or anxious on a lower dose of medication.

There have been multiple reports suggesting that some babies whose moms used antidepressants in the third trimester experience a "withdrawal" after delivery. What has been observed is a time-limited (a few hours to a few days) syndrome of mild symptoms including fussiness, trouble eating or sleeping, or more need for medical monitoring. There is no evidence of long-term effects. It's important that you and your partner understand this potential reaction, so if your baby is more fussy, you can feel reassured that it will resolve. And this temporary situation is certainly preferable to you suffering unnecessarily with depression during pregnancy when medication could have helped.

A few reports suggest that babies might be at risk for earlier delivery if the mother is taking antidepressants. It is certainly difficult to separate out what might be the effects of stress, depression, and anxiety (which can possibly cause an earlier delivery) as opposed to the effect of a medication, since women usually do not take medication without a good reason during pregnancy (depression and anxiety being good reasons). One scary, but isolated, report showed that a serious but very rare lung condition might be more common in women who use SSRIs in late pregnancy. An important thing to keep in mind, however, is that most studies in this area have included too few patients. In addition, these studies do

About Paxil

If paroxetine (Paxil) has worked for you in the past, then it's absolutely among the best choices for you during pregnancy. And if you're on paroxetine and find yourself pregnant, don't abruptly stop taking it. Pregnancy is not a good time for medication "tryouts." This is not the appropriate time to experiment with other medications when you already know something works for you. However, if you've never been on an antidepressant before, your doctor will probably choose a different one for you to try first, considering the recent concerns about possible fetal heart defects and withdrawal symptoms. These concerns may, in the end, be shown to be based on something real—or not. But at this point, there is enough confusion that if you haven't tried something else that has worked for you, another SSRI will probably be the preferred first choice.

not adequately take into account the consequences of not taking the antidepressant when needed—in other words, the problems of an untreated psychiatric disorder—which also affect pregnancy and the baby's growth and development. The most scary information always makes the best headlines, and health-care providers who know the least about this area of research are understandably the ones who are most vulnerable to misinterpreting it.

A third category of antidepressants, monoamine oxidase inhibitors (MAOIs), such as phenelzine (Nardil) and tranylcypromine (Parnate), may cause birth defects and are not considered to be safe during pregnancy.

Note of caution: If you have a personal or family history of bipolar disorder, you should be monitored extra carefully if you're taking an antidepressant—even if you're also taking a mood stabilizer. An antidepressant can increase your risk of a manic episode.

Don't Play the Milligram Game

When you're prescribed a medication during pregnancy, understand that you may need more of the medication than you may have needed before you became pregnant. This doesn't mean you're more ill. You're simply metabolizing differently— there's more blood volume surging through your system, so you need more medication to get the same effect.

ANTIANXIETY MEDICATIONS

Anxiety is a frequent symptom of depression in pregnancy. At first you may only be aware of the anxiety and not the depression. Sometimes after the anxiety decreases, the depression under the surface is revealed and needs to be handled. Benzodiazepines are medications used to help reduce anxiety, either during the day or at night to help with insomnia. These medications can be quite useful and are taken on an "as-needed" basis, unlike antidepressants, which require that you take a pill every day. For instance, if you feel a panic attack coming on, it's nice to know that a bit of the medication you have in your purse will take the panic away in a matter of minutes.

Some of the medications included in this category are loraze-pam (Ativan), diazepam (Valium), clonazepam (Klonopin), and alprazolam (Xanax). These medications are potentially addictive, but when they're taken appropriately and not abused, this is rarely an issue. I have found in my practice (and my colleagues agree) that, in general, pregnant women are trying so hard not to take any medication that the opposite tends to happen. In other words, often these women need to be coaxed to take one of these medications—their anxiety (the reason they need the medication in the first place) makes them worry too much about taking it. Sometimes doctors prescribe only a few of these pills at a time since they're trying to be cautious. Ironically, this can cause you to have extra anxiety since you're anticipating running out of what's helping your anxiety! But the doctors I work the most closely with feel comfortable prescribing small doses to pregnant and breast-feeding mothers for months, if necessary. Often antianxiety medications help a pregnant woman out of crisis until the antidepressant (or other method of treatment) kicks in, and then the antianxiety med isn't needed anymore. It all depends on your individual situation. Interestingly, the antidepressants that affect serotonin are generally all excellent at helping to alleviate anxiety, but it does take a while (usually weeks) for the benefits to be felt, so sometimes a short-term plan for a benzodiazepine is needed if the anxiety is severe.

> Often antianxiety medications help a pregnant woman out of crisis until the antidepressant (or other method of treatment) kicks in, and then the antianxiety med isn't needed anymore.

There had been some early reports of an increase in the risk for cleft lip or palate when those drugs are used in the first trimester. However, not all studies have supported an association between benzodiazepines and any birth defects. Ideally, benzodiazepines should be avoided in the first trimester (while organs are forming) and at the very end of pregnancy (to avoid the baby having withdrawal effects of the medication at the time of delivery). However, untreated anxiety can certainly be incapacitating for the mother and can increase risks for her baby as well. So if she needs it, she should take it.

Not too long ago, the media also announced that these babies whose moms had benzodiazepines in their system can go through "withdrawal" upon birth. When you think about someone going through withdrawal, what do you envision? Probably an adult coming off heroin—horrible pain, violent shaking, vomiting, and so on, right? Well, get rid of that picture in your head. Here's what the "withdrawal" looks like: Some of these newborns experience some jitteriness, irritability, and sleep disturbances, and these issues resolve on their own as the drug leaves the baby's system. If you are taking a benzodiazepine at the time of delivery, make sure your OB and the baby's pediatrician know so that your baby will be observed for any of those temporary symptoms. If you're breast-feeding while taking any of these medications, watch the baby for extra sleepiness, lack of energy to suck, or low energy in general (which is hard to tell since newborns sleep a lot anyway). These drugs have been on the market for over forty years, and there hasn't been any evidence to suggest that they have long-term negative effects on the child.

Note of caution: If you have a history of substance abuse, you may be nervous about taking a potentially addictive medication. You should seriously discuss with your doctor the medications that are least likely to cause relapse with substance abuse. When there are not other good alternatives, remember that it's better to properly and appropriately take a prescribed medication than it is to self-medicate. Always make sure to let your doctor know about your history and take care to stick to the prescribed amount of the medication.

Testing Baby's Health and Yours during Pregnancy

If you're taking lithium or paroxetine (Paxil), or for any reason you're worried about your baby's heart development (if there is a family history of cardiovascular defects, for instance), you should know about fetal echocardiography, a noninvasive ultrasound technique that looks at your baby's heart structure and its function. The direction of blood flow is assessed using in-color techniques. For almost all babies the test results are normal, and this will be extremely reassuring for you. This test can typically be done at the time of a routine ultrasound.

If you're on a medication that has a risk of teratogenicity (can cause birth defects)—for example, an anticonvulsant—you might want to ask for a Level II or "high-risk" ultrasound, a step beyond the routine screening ultrasound during which an expert in this field takes a very close look at the baby's growth and development. It's essential to have this high-risk ultrasound when you're taking medications such as valproate and carbamazepine, which are mood stabilizers and anticonvulsants. These medications carry the small but serious risk of neural tube defects (birth defects in the brain and spinal cord). Some obstetricians will automatically order this test for you, but you may need to ask for it.

All pregnant women are routinely screened for gestational diabetes. If you're taking an atypical antipsychotic medication, be certain to mention this to your OB since those meds are associated with an increased risk of elevated blood glucose. Your OB might choose to monitor you even more closely in this situation, which would be a good thing.

Thyroid problems are common in women in general, and during pregnancy and postpartum especially (10 percent of postpartum moms have a thyroid disorder). Thyroid dysfunction can cause similar symptoms as depression—especially in the case of hypothyroidism. In addition, hypothyroidism is a side effect of lithium treatment. Luckily, thyroid function tests are easy to get and just involve taking a bit of blood.

In pregnancy, there are very serious effects of untreated hypothyroidism (too little thyroid hormone) for the baby, so it's very important that your thyroid is tested, especially if you're depressed or taking lithium. The good news is that it's easily treated with thyroid hormone supplementation. Women who have thyroid problems should be

> *monitored extra carefully during pregnancy and postpartum. Too little thyroid hormone can make a woman fatigued, feel slowed down, and depressed; too much can make her anxious, panicky, jittery, and too energized (in a bad way).*
>
> *Anemia can also contribute to fatigue. A blood count is an easy test that is usually completed during pregnancy at least once, and your doctor may suggest iron if your red blood cell count is low. If you know you have had anemia before, mention it to your doctor, and ask if you should take iron supplements. Some foods are also rich in iron, such as leafy greens.*

SLEEP AIDS

Sleep is a huge issue during pregnancy and new motherhood. Sometimes even when your environment is set up for you to get good sleep, your body and mind won't allow it. It might be an inability to fall asleep, to stay asleep, or you may have early-morning wakening (way too early). Ideally, medications prescribed just for sleep can be used short-term and just as a backup when nonmedication strategies like relaxation techniques do not work. You should make sure to avoid caffeine and other stimulants (which are often found in surprising places, such as energy drinks or bars, or even supplements) and employ soothing strategies to promote restfulness before bed, such as the right kind of exercise (although not right before bed), or reading "fluff." If some of these techniques feel too overwhelming and not possible for you to do right now, don't worry. Just do the best you can. If your difficulty sleeping is caused by anxiety, I'd be willing to bet you probably won't be able to use meditation—even if this technique has always been helpful to you before. Taking deep breaths can be useful, but attempting to calm your mind for meditation will probably be futile and frustrating while you're dealing with anxiety. Cognitive behavioral and other psychotherapy strategies are often extremely effective. Remember, medication is an important part of your regimen if you need it, but you want to avoid it when you can. Many sleep aids are heavily marketed, and direct-to-consumer advertisements are everywhere we look, but the safety of many of these medications during pregnancy has not been well established.

> Make sure that you do not take a sleep aid that has a pain management or allergy medicine you do not need, as many over-the-counter preparations are "cocktails," and you want to minimize unnecessary medications during pregnancy.

Your doctor might want you to try an over-the-counter medication before a prescription medication. Make sure, however, that you do not take a sleep aid that has a pain management or allergy medicine you do not need, as many over-the-counter preparations are "cocktails," and you want to minimize unnecessary medications during pregnancy. Sleep aids, including medications such as zolpidem (Ambien) and the benzodiazepines, help with insomnia, although safety has not been adequately assessed for many of these during pregnancy. Tricyclic antidepressants with sedative effects, such as amitriptyline (Elavil), trazodone

(Desyrel), and nortriptyline (Pamelor), are often used as sleep aids as well.

If nothing works for your insomnia, make sure your doctor knows. One of your medications might be contributing to the sleep problem. For instance, sometimes an SSRI can make insomnia worse, so your doctor may suggest taking it at a different time of day and the problem will go away. Another reason to tell your doctor if your insomnia doesn't decrease is because your diagnosis might need to be reevaluated to make sure you are receiving the best treatment.

Note: Anecdotally, the sleep glasses I discuss in chapter 7 have often worked beautifully with pregnant women and helped them avoid sleep aids or get off them.

MOOD STABILIZERS

Mood stabilizers are mainly prescribed to individuals with bipolar disorder (also called manic depression), and since this disorder usually includes episodes of both mania and depression, more than one medication is usually necessary. Sometimes mood stabilizers are used in conjunction with antidepressants. Lithium, anticonvulsants, and atypical antipsychotic medications are frequently prescribed mood stabilizers. If your doctor prescribes an "antipsychotic," it's not necessarily because he thinks you're psychotic.

Lithium used to be considered contraindicated during pregnancy, but newer updated information demonstrates it is a reasonable option for pregnant women who respond well to it. In fact, stopping it increases the risk of mood episodes in pregnant and postpartum women. There is a very low risk of a very rare cardiac condition with its use in the first trimester. At the time of your ultrasound, however, you can get a fetal echocardiogram, an ultrasound technique that looks at your baby's heart and its function. This is a noninvasive test and can decrease your anxiety if you are concerned about this risk. Note that lithium is not recommended for use during breast-feeding. Pregnant women taking lithium should have their lithium levels monitored regularly, as in late pregnancy their blood levels might drop, leaving them more vulnerable to mood episodes. Also, lithium increases the risk of hypothyroidism, and maternal hypothyroidism has very serious risks for the baby, so thyroid tests should also be done during pregnancy. Not all obstetricians will routinely check this, so make sure you ask for it if you use lithium during pregnancy. (For whatever reason, if you do have a hypothyroid condition, you may be prescribed levothyroxine [Synthroid]. Make sure that you do not take this medication at the same time of the day as you take a calcium supplement. The calcium will decrease your body's ability to absorb the thyroid supplement.)

Valproate (Depakote) has the highest risk in pregnancy of any psychiatric medication, with a reported 1 to 5 percent risk of neural tube defects when used in the very early first trimester. Thus, it should not be taken in early pregnancy. Interestingly, the reverse is true for these two medications in breast-feeding. Depakote is considered low risk during breast-feeding and is approved by the American Academy of Pediatrics (AAP). Newer anticonvulsants do not appear to have the same level of risk in pregnancy as valproate. While there have been some reports of increased risk of cleft palate with lamotrigine, it is commonly used in bipolar disorder to prevent depressive episodes. More research on these medications is needed.

ANTIPSYCHOTICS

For women who have psychotic disorders, the danger of an untreated illness is extremely high. Psychosis by definition includes impairment in judgment, and a psychotic woman cannot take the best care of herself that she and her baby deserve. In fact, the danger is so high that if she is postpartum with a new baby, or has other children in the home, they should be considered at great risk for harm. The woman should be hospitalized, and if that's not possible, another adult should be with her at all times, never leaving her alone or alone with her child(ren) until she is more stable.

Antipsychotic medications used in pregnancy include atypical antipsychotics (used also as mood stabilizers). So far, studies have not demonstrated an increased risk of birth defects with these medications. Older medications such as haloperidol may also be reasonable options for pregnant women. These are the same antipsychotic medications that are used when a breast-feeding mom has postpartum psychosis.

A Word about Psychosis

Very different from depression, a woman in a psychotic state is not in our reality. She is hallucinating—seeing, hearing, or feeling things that others don't who are in the same room. She also may be having bizarre thoughts. Typically, a woman who has a psychotic episode in pregnancy has a history of psychosis. Psychosis is quite rare in pregnancy unless the woman has a chronic psychotic disorder (such as schizophrenia or bipolar disorder with psychotic features), but when it does occur, it's always considered to be a medical emergency—it's very dangerous. You never can predict what's going through her mind at any given moment and what delusional thought may prompt her to harm herself or her child. Hospitalization is always advised so she can be kept safe (and therefore her baby is kept safe). Antipsychotic medications are used to treat her, and electroconvulsive therapy (ECT) is commonly administered. Although this sounds extreme to some, ECT isn't scary or painful. Although in the movies ECT is depicted as a gruesome procedure, the modern-day process is very humane. A short-duration general anesthesia is used, and the treatment itself takes only seconds. It is generally considered safe for the baby. Based on a large body of literature, few complications have been reported, except for the woman's short-term memory loss of the hours right before and right after the ECT (occasionally her memory loss lasts longer). ECT is also considered a good treatment choice for severely depressed pregnant women. It has about an 80 percent success rate. There is still a great deal of misinformation about this treatment, but now it is considered to be a very important and lifesaving treatment by experts in the field internationally.

Testing Drugs on Pregnant Women

Drugs are not tested on pregnant women, as the research issues are complicated. No one wants to withhold an effective treatment from a suffering pregnant woman, but at the same time, no one wants to expose babies to a possible risk from medication either. So scientific, controlled studies are not available for medication, and I doubt they ever will be. The safety data and the relapse data during pregnancy that are available are based on the outcomes when women chose to take or not take medication.

Sometimes data have emerged quite accidentally. For example, most of the drug companies have what's known as voluntary registries, where people taking medications can report any side effects or positive benefits. Women in studies were sometimes asked not to get pregnant during the study since no one wanted the liability. But since the women felt better on the medications, they started resuming normal activities, one of which was sex. Since they were still on the medications when they got pregnant, the women reported their experiences with the medications while pregnant.

Treat to Wellness

Your doctor should treat you with enough medication so you feel well. She should prescribe the lowest dosage necessary for you to feel like you—not just to take the edge off. Inadequate treatment leads to a bad prognosis—often chronic depression. Again, there's plenty you can do to help treat your depression naturally, but the point is, get fully treated.

Should I Believe the Media?

With little exception, the media thrives on negativity. I always suggest to those I care about that they not watch the news— not only if they're suffering with depression or anxiety, but all the time. I'm a very informed person, but I haven't watched the news in over a decade. The news is anxiety producing and depressing. The media is interested in ratings—whatever people will watch, that's what they provide—and fear sells. On any station, at any given time, you'll hear and see hype and sensationalism. We are continuously bombarded with various types of warnings that can scare us unnecessarily. When it's announced that a rare form of illness is wafting through the air, a big earthquake is coming within the next few years, risks of terrorist attacks are imminent, and so on, how does that help the public on a practical level? The answer is, it doesn't. There isn't anything practical to do with that information—it just gets you worked up into an anxious state if you're not careful. This helps no one, and instead hurts us and those around us.

> No matter what you hear from the media— whether TV, radio, or print—check with a medical practitioner you trust. Your doctor is trained to discern what's important to pay attention to and what you should ignore.

So when a scary message comes over the airwaves about a particular medication that you're taking or thinking of taking, it's essential that you regard the report with a healthy degree of skepticism and consult with your practitioner. The wording of these reports is purposefully crafted to shock the listener, so that you'll keep tuning in to that particular show. Rarely is the whole truth given, since that isn't what gets ratings.

It's important to find out what "research" they are talking about. Are the researchers affiliated with a particular drug company, or are they independent researchers or competitors? Does the news report sound "antipsychiatry" in general? What can really be concluded from the information gathered—what's the real scoop, without the hype? Whatever you do, never quit an antidepressant or any psychiatric medication cold turkey. No matter what you hear from the media—whether TV, radio, or print—check with a medical practitioner you trust. Your doctor is trained to discern what's important to pay attention to and what you should ignore.

Sensational and unusual stories (especially the negative ones) make good sound bites—they catch attention, which is the media's intention. The real discussion of risks and benefits regarding medication is too long and complicated for the media's interest and typical attention span. Too often stories are not comprehensive and don't show the whole picture. Also, a particular story may not pertain to your situation at all, but it's reported in a way that can make you think it does.

One example of misrepresented data that did quite a lot of harm was regarding hormone replacement therapy (HRT). Since this isn't the topic of the book, I won't elaborate here, but suffice it to say that the way the media portrayed the research, omitting key facts, women everywhere became terrified that they were giving themselves cancer and stopped their HRT. This caused considerable problems—both physical and emotional.

Never stop taking your medication without speaking to your doctor first. Stopping antidepressants suddenly can cause many problems. Pregnant women with bipolar disorder who stop taking their medication have a 50 percent relapse rate in the first three months and a 70 percent relapse rate by six months. (These statistics differ among studies, but the point is, sudden discontinuation of the medication causes problems.)

Not too long ago, the FDA announced that paroxetine (Paxil) may cause heart problems for the baby when a pregnant woman takes it during the first trimester, switching it from category C to D. This threw the medical community into a tizzy. Psychiatrists weren't sure where this information originated, and if true, they weren't sure if this meant that all of the SSRIs may cause problems or just this one. Overnight, it seemed, treating depressed pregnant women became even more complicated, and psychiatrists felt less confident to prescribe. This announcement was not based on research that was reviewed or published, so it was not easily available to the medical community.

A study recently published in the *American Journal of Psychiatry* reports that there is no association between paroxetine and heart malformations, and doctors have yet to actually see any study performed with animals that supports the FDA's announcement or the original research upon which this scary announcement was based. Doctors learned nothing about how the research was conducted or how the conclusions were made. It's been hidden and private. The Paxil announcement was not helpful either to medical professionals or to the public. Although no one knows just what to do with the Paxil information, two reliable resources for checking the safety of medications for women in pregnancy are Motherisk (www.motherisk.org, which is the same organization that conducted the recent paroxetine study) and OTIS (www.otispregnancy.org).

Not the Time to Switch

One thing that's known for sure—if a particular medication is working for you, and there's no clear reason to go off it, stay on it. Even if another medication has more safety data behind it, during pregnancy, when you're extra vulnerable, is not the time to experiment. The same is true if you're lining up a plan of action for yourself just in case you need it. If you've tried a medication before and it doesn't work well for you, don't go on it simply because it's used more often in pregnancy. You need to use what works. Remember that depression and anxiety cross the placenta and can affect the development of your baby's brain. Depression in pregnancy is associated with low birth weight, preterm delivery, babies who are small for their gestational age, and other birth complications. Even minor depression may affect the fetus. Severe anxiety in pregnancy can cause constriction of the blood vessels in the placenta and heightened startle response in your newborn, and your baby may be harder to soothe. If you don't want to use natural healing methods or they don't seem to be effective for you, do whatever it takes to feel normal. "Toughing it out" is never a good idea.

For example, when my client Fran first called me, she was thoroughly confused, upset, anxious, and depressed. For the last two years, she and her husband, Greg, had tried everything to get pregnant, even flying to the East Coast from California to go through an expensive experimental program in the hope of increasing their chances of fertility. To their delight, it worked. Fran had a history of prenatal anxiety, which she had mistakenly not planned for this time around. She had thought that since she was so happy and excited about the pregnancy that she wouldn't be hit with anxiety this time. This is a common and understandable (but very untrue) way of thinking. When you feel great, it's almost impossible to anticipate feeling bad again. The opposite is also true. When you're feeling anxious or depressed, it's very difficult to imagine yourself ever feeling happy again. This was exactly what happened to Fran. Since Fran had not told the psychiatrist who had previously treated her for two pre-natal anxiety disorders with her first two children that she was pregnant again, she had no medical plan of action. Her wishful thinking was naïve. She was actually very high risk, having experienced not only one, but two anxiety disorders in pregnancy before becoming pregnant this time.

She was not in therapy either, which should have been part of her pre-pregnancy plan. By the time she was hit with severe anxiety, about three weeks into the pregnancy, she was having thoughts such as, "What was I thinking? My life was wonderful before getting pregnant. I should have just been happy with my two kids and not risked this horrible illness again. I know Greg and I were trying hard for this pregnancy, but we hadn't thought it out. I can't handle this pregnancy. I could never handle another baby. I made a horrible mistake!" She doubted ever really wanting to get pregnant, even though rationally she knew how badly she had craved another child. She was panic stricken, and she obsessed on whether or not to abort, fluctuating back and forth with her decision for a few weeks. Her husband was leaving the decision up to her, and he too was conflicted. Although he was disappointed at the thought of losing the opportunity to have this child, he also saw how ill his wife was and wanted her and their lives to return to normal.

The first time Fran went to the doctor's office to terminate the pregnancy, she left right before the procedure began, still unsure about what to do. Then she decided to go through with the abortion and did so. It was one week after the abortion that she contacted me.

Fran relayed to me—through a combination of tears, anger, guilt, confusion, and extreme remorse—that she desperately needed help. She was beside herself with myriad powerful emotions. I requested that Greg be part of this first session since I felt his perspective might be helpful. In short, after the abortion, Fran experienced an immediate relief since she believed the pregnancy was the root of the problem, and therefore, when the pregnancy was gone, her life would be normal. Far from it. About two days later she was hit with a depression and severe grief about the loss. She wasn't feeling the anxiety anymore, so she was able to rationally process information about what had happened. The reality of the events and feelings that led up to the abortion was setting in. Fran needed compassion for herself, information about what had happened in her brain chemistry when she was pregnant, and the understanding of what she had badly needed but hadn't received when she was going through the anxiety. Although this was an extremely painful time for her, Fran was eventually able to forgive herself and realize that she had done the best she could with the information she had at the time. And, although it wouldn't erase what happened, if she and Greg chose to, they could move ahead with another pregnancy with a solid and realistic plan of action this time.

Over-the-Counter Meds

Many over-the-counter drugs can be used during pregnancy under a physician's supervision, but some are known to be unsafe. If you're pregnant, possibly pregnant, or nursing, consult with your doctor before taking anything. For instance, aspirin should be avoided in the last three months of pregnancy because it may cause problems in utero for the baby or complications during delivery. Ibuprofen is also not recommended during the third trimester. As I discussed in chapter 7, just because something is natural doesn't make it safe. The same goes for over-the-counter medicines.

Medication and Breast-feeding

I'm often asked if taking a medication in pregnancy will prohibit breast-feeding. With only one exception, the current wisdom states that if it's okay in pregnancy, it's okay when breast-feeding, since now the baby's own system is filtering the medication, and the baby receives much less of the medication than he or she did in utero. The exception is lithium, a mood stabilizer used primarily for treating bipolar illness. While lithium is used in pregnancy but not breast-feeding, the opposite is true for Depakote, another mood stabilizer. Depakote has up to a 5 percent risk of neural tube defects when used in pregnancy, but it's accepted by the American Academy of Pediatrics for breast-feeding moms. Lithium has a very low risk (0.01–0.2 percent) of Ebstein's anomaly (treatable heart defect) when taken in the first trimester, but it's much safer than a manic episode. Although this is a higher rate as compared to the general population not taking lithium, the risk for this anomaly is extremely small with or without lithium. In weighing the risks of an untreated bipolar disorder as compared with taking lithium, most women clearly need treatment. With untreated bipolar disorder, the scary risks of having a manic episode or a major depressive episode—both of which are dangerous for the mother and baby—are much greater than the tiny risk of taking the medication.

Key Points

- *Mood and anxiety disorders are medical conditions, and there is no shame in receiving treatment for them. Ideally, medication should be prescribed as part of a comprehensive treatment plan that also includes therapy.*

- *Research on medication in pregnancy is constantly evolving, which is why it is so important to see a doctor who has the necessary expertise and dedication to stay up-to-date on the latest findings.*

- *Two reliable resources for checking the safety of medications during pregnancy are www.motherisk.org and www.otispregnancy.org.*

- *If a medication is working for you, and there is no clear reason to go off it, then stay on it— pregnancy is not the time to experiment.*

Chapter 7

NATURAL AND EMERGING TREATMENTS

Even though some professionals may have their preferences and lean toward either prescribing medication
or using natural healing modalities, most practitioners
today are open-minded and genuinely interested in helping their clients and patients recover, using whatever
methods work well for them. Hopefully, your practitioner
is one of these. If not, I suggest you find someone who
is. My belief has always been that one should use whatever combination of treatments works to reach 100 percent wellness—as long as it's safe. Your body chemistry,
beliefs, and comfort levels regarding various treatments
are different from the next woman's, so an individual plan
is important.

I am a believer in "natural whenever possible," but
this does not in any way imply that I'm against medication when needed. Nor do I believe that just because a
treatment is natural, it's necessarily more effective or better. Women have been asking me more and more if I can
help them avoid medication, and while I never promise
to do that, over the last twenty years I've often seen fast

and dramatic changes in those who use natural methods. The body is meant to heal itself, and when given a fighting chance, that's what tends to happen. With a comprehensive plan of action that includes sleep, excellent nutrition, emotional and physical support, therapy, plus various combinations of the treatments listed in this chapter, women often show great improvement. Sometimes medication is needed in addition, and sometimes it's not. What's most important is that the woman feels like herself again.

It's exciting that many of the methods discussed in this chapter are showing promise in the field of maternal mental health (even though some of the natural treatments are not new at all—they have been used effectively for thousands of years). Since women are increasingly showing great interest in exploring all their options, it's important that these emerging treatments be covered in this book.

Complementary and Alternative Medicine

Unfortunately, and often incorrectly, many people assume the term *alternative treatment* implies that it's unproven or off-the-wall. For that reason I frequently use the term *emerging treatment, meaning it's a legitimate treatment currently in the process of being formally tested.* However, *alternative* does have its place, especially in the context of Complementary and Alternative Medicine (CAM). Some emerging treatments can sometimes be used in place of prescription medication (referred to as "alternative"), and some emerging treatments can be used only in addition to medication or alternative treatment (referred to as "complementary").

Be Wary of the Internet

Especially regarding the topic of Complementary and Alternative Medicine (CAM) treatments, be careful about trying to find information about them on the Internet (and if you're anxious, stay away from the Internet in general). When you search for CAM methods, many bogus sites spewing nonsense will pop up. Most often they're trying to sell you something that won't work. Bottom line is, it's hard to tell what to trust and what to ignore, so I suggest you go to NCCAM's Web site, http://nccam. nih.gov. This federally funded site offers current research and reliable information about complementary and alternative medicine.

Now that CAM treatments have become so popular, more attention is being paid to them. For example, the National Center for Complementary and Alternative Medicine (NCCAM) scientifically explores emerging healing methods and educates professionals and the public about their effectiveness. While there's not much clinical experimental evidence about CAM treatments for pregnancy (unfortunately, clinical studies are expensive and take years to perform, so they are generally only carried out when the treatment will be profitable), it's still appropriate and helpful to discuss them. One can always argue that until a method is tested specifically in any subgroup (like pregnant women) it should not be recommended, but when the methods are not showing any ill effects and are proving to be quite effective, it would be doing women a disservice to ignore them, causing unnecessary suffering for those who may benefit from knowing about them. I will provide you with a few of these methods in this chapter. Some of them have more research to date than others, but additional research is currently ongoing.

Integrative Medicine

A few psychotherapists and medical doctors feel threatened about the modes of treatment outlined in this chapter, since these healing methods are different from what they've been taught. Since the public is very interested in using CAM treatments, however, these practitioners will need to adapt, or their practices will eventually die off. Intelligent and open-minded medical and mental-health practitioners are the majority, fortunately, and they are opening up to information regarding these modalities. Many practitioners are even specifically studying these methods in order to incorporate them into their practices and help their patients even more. This type of medical professional is practicing what is called integrative medicine, a term that is used to reflect a style of treatment that's open to all options that have proven effective, whether conventional or alternative. Integrative medicine takes into account the whole person—body, mind, and spirit—and makes use of conventional and alternative therapies that have research to back them up. Psychiatrists and other M.D.s need to be educated about CAM modalities so they can discuss them with their patients. (I hope the term *alternative* will eventually disappear in this context entirely since, in actuality, a treatment is a treatment.)

The following treatments are listed in alphabetical order. All of these categories have at least some research behind them demonstrating effectiveness in treating mood disorders. It is not an exhaustive list by any means, but you'll get a feel for some of the best and most commonly used natural treatments out there. To explore a wider list of options, you can visit NCCAM's Web site, http://nccam.nih.gov.

Choosing a Practitioner

When deciding on a practitioner for a treatment that you've chosen, there are a few factors to consider. If the particular discipline you want to try has licensing requirements for its professionals, make sure he or she is licensed. Word of mouth is the best reference, but if you're not sure about the source, ask for references from the practitioner and follow up on them. Most importantly, whoever you choose to work with should have the training and expertise (actual experience) that's required. And, of course, you should feel comfortable with the person and have a good rapport. This will foster good communication, which is necessary for the best working relationships.

Here's a rundown of some of the most popular categories of practitioners so you can differentiate who's who:

***Medical doctors (M.D.s)** are the most well known, since they are typically the professionals who deliver most of the health care people receive. Most excellent M.D.s these days are proficient at* *delivering not only traditional Western medicine but also are open-minded to Complementary and Alternative Medicine (CAM).*

Naturopaths (N.D.s) *are practitioners of alternative medicine who earn a degree after four years of rigorous training. In the United States, each state determines whether the naturopath can prescribe medication (and what types they're allowed to prescribe). In addition to alternative treatments, naturopaths are keenly focused on nutrition.*

Chiropractors (D.C.s) *are mainly focused on the spine, adjusting spinal misalignments so patients can experience healing. When the flow of nerve impulses is restored with the adjustment, the body can self-regulate and heal itself. Chiropractors often prescribe supplements of various kinds to their patients.*

Osteopaths (D.O.s), *like chiropractors, are focused primarily on the musculoskeletal system, which includes the nerves, muscles, and bones. D.O.s are known for taking the whole person—both their physical and psychological needs—into account when administering treatment. Like an M.D., a D.O. is licensed for the unlimited practice of medicine in every state in the United States, which means that a D.O. can prescribe medications and surgeries, plus any other treatment or medical test.*

Acupuncturists *(usually listed as L.Ac., but there are many variations) are used for many different conditions, including infertility, depression, and pain. Acupuncture can take many years of* *study. If you can find a practitioner who obtained his license in China, that's the best, but the United States does have licensing boards for acupuncturists. Check with the National Certification Commission for Acupuncture and Oriental Medicine (NCCAOM) at www.nccaom.org or the American Board of Medical Acupuncture at www.dabma.org to make sure the practitioner is board certified.*

Massage therapists (L.M.T.s) *may be trained in a variety of massage techniques, and an experienced massage therapist can be quite helpful for your body and mind during pregnancy. Your massage therapist should be certified; a good organization for checking certification is the National Certification Board for Therapeutic Massage and Bodywork (www.ncbtmb.com). The American Massage Therapy Association (www.amtamassage.org) recommends that you ask the following questions before you decide to work with the practitioner:*

- *Are you licensed to practice massage?*

- *Are you nationally certified in therapeutic massage and bodywork?*

- *Where did you receive your massage therapy training?*

- *Do you belong to the American Massage Therapy Association?*

During pregnancy, it's especially important that your massage therapist is experienced and knowledgeable in working with pregnant women. This is a specialty for two reasons: Certain positions are obviously more comfortable and safe, like lying on your side instead of your stomach, and particular areas of your body should be manipulated very carefully or avoided altogether. Those massage therapists who are excellent working with pregnant women are often also great with new moms who have loose ligaments and sore, healing muscles.

Herbalists *are known for treating the whole person and not just the symptom of an illness. For instance, each person who consults with the same herbalist for the same condition may leave the office with completely different prescriptions. Your herbalist should be registered with an organization called the National Institute of Medical Herbalists (nimh.org.uk).*

Acupuncture

Acupuncture is an ancient method of healing that uses fine needles in specific points on the body. According to Chinese medicine, acupuncture works by altering the flow of energy along various meridians of the body, thereby correcting imbalances. Acupuncture increases melatonin, which reduces anxiety and insomnia. The World Health Organization (WHO) now recognizes acupuncture as a complementary treatment for 104 conditions, one of which is depression.

In an experiment at Beijing University of Chinese Medicine, patients were assigned to two groups: an acupuncture group and a medication group. The acupuncture group received acupuncture treatment six times a week for six weeks, and the medication group received a daily dose of amitriptyline (a tricyclic antidepressant), beginning with 25 milligrams and increasing to 300 milligrams over six weeks. The result was that there was no significant difference between the two groups. Both groups improved equally.

The study concluded that "acupuncture is as effective a treatment option for depression as amitriptyline," but while the results are impressive, this won't necessarily be true for everyone. And, no matter what, therapy is needed whether you're using acupuncture, medication, or a combination of both.

The bottom line is, high-quality research with adequate numbers of participants are lacking for acupuncture. Plus, of the studies that have been done, the results regarding major depression are mixed.

ACUPUNCTURE IN PREGNANCY

Acupuncture is showing promise as a safe, effective treatment for both depression and anxiety in pregnancy, but more studies are needed. Pregnant women must be cautious and only work with highly skilled practitioners. The reason for this is that some acupuncture points may cause uterine stimulation and increase the ripening of the cervix, speeding labor. In a study of depressed pregnant women, those who received acupuncture improved more than the control group (no treatment) or the massage group.

In a study from Dr. Rachel Manber and her colleagues at Stanford University, acupuncture was used with a group of sixty-one depressed pregnant women. Sixty-nine percent of the women improved from the acupuncture, a rate that is comparable to the 50 to 70 percent improvement rates in clinical studies of other standard treatments for depression. The study suggests that acupuncture may be as effective as interpersonal psychotherapy and cognitive-behavioral therapy (see chapter 3 for a description of these talk therapies). In addition, acupuncture for depression in pregnancy significantly reduces the rate of postpartum depression. Again, it's worth repeating that although acupuncture may relieve the physiological symptoms of depression, which is wonderful, it does not in any way replace what psychotherapy provides. Therapy teaches life skills—stress management, role adjustments, communication, and much more—which help in your present life as well as decrease the risk of a future episode. Acupuncture does not teach these skills. Therefore, acupuncture plus psychotherapy can be a powerful combination.

> **Acupuncture plus psychotherapy can be a powerful combination.**

Energy Psychology

Energy-based techniques such as EFT (Emotional Freedom Technique) and EMDR (Eye Movement Desensitization and Reprocessing) are powerful and noninvasive. The Association for Comprehensive Energy Psychology (ACEP) and the International Society for the Study of Subtle Energies and Energy Medicine (ISSSEEM) train licensed medical and mental-health practitioners in the use of these methods. EFT, a simple technique that requires no equipment except your own hands, has been successful in thousands of clinical cases. It

EFT has been successful in thousands of clinical cases. Many M.D.s (including psychiatrists) and psychotherapists use it with great success to help patients with depression, obsessive-compulsive disorder, and other mood and anxiety disorders.

happens to be a personal favorite of mine. Many M.D.s (including psychiatrists) and psychotherapists use it with great success to help patients with depression, obsessive-compulsive disorder, and other mood and anxiety disorders. EFT is not yet in the standard medical literature, and the field needs more formal research. As you're reading this, however, clinical trials are being conducted in the United States. For more information go to www.eftinternational.com.

To date, research is lacking to support the use of EMDR for depression and other mood disorders, but it has been proven quite effective for posttraumatic stress disorder (PTSD). In 2004 the American Psychiatric Association reported that EMDR received the highest level of recommendation, which means that it has the best scientific proof for effectiveness. Also in 2004, the Department of Veterans Affairs and the Department of Defense put EMDR in the A category, which states, "strongly recommended for the treatment of trauma."

ENERGY PSYCHOLOGY IN PREGNANCY
There have been no ill effects reported that I'm aware of when using energy psychology techniques. These are noninvasive techniques, and they are regarded as harmless by the medical

practitioners who use them with their patients. There have been no formal studies regarding their use in pregnancy.

Liz's Story

I feel some shame and guilt in writing this piece because I have had so much more help to recover from my PPD than most women have. I have had several therapists, a psychiatrist, an acupressurist, postpartum doulas, a full-time nanny, a sleep consultant, no job to go to, and a husband who does a great deal of child care. I am very grateful for everything it took to get to where I am now, and I hope that many women, even if they don't have all the help I did, will find my experiences helpful.

I was always afraid of being pregnant and giving birth. I loved babies and kids, though, so I thought maybe I'd just adopt. But then as I got older, I started to think I'd like to try to get pregnant, despite my fears. I met my husband when I was almost thirty-seven and married just after turning thirty-eight. We were in a hurry to marry so we could try to get pregnant, but we quickly found out that I was already too old; I had "decreased ovarian reserve," meaning my eggs were too old. This was a shock, even though I knew that women's fertility wanes after age thirty-five. Our reproductive endocrinologist suggested using donor eggs, which I had never imagined or thought about, but it seemed like a good option. The baby could have my husband's genes, I could be pregnant and breast-feed, and we could choose a donor whose genetics seemed like a good match for me.

We found a great donor match very quickly, and I went through IVF with the donor eggs and got pregnant. I had just turned thirty-nine. I was happy to be pregnant but was often anxious about how the pregnancy was going. Did spotting mean I was miscarrying? I lay on the couch, searched through my many books on pregnancy, and called the OB for reassurance. Did those contractions mean preterm labor? I rushed to the hospital to get it checked out. My husband was annoyed and frustrated whenever I got overly anxious. I just wanted reassurance and for him to help me sort out whether there was anything to worry about. But he became frustrated with me when he couldn't help me with my anxiety. The marital tensions made me feel even more anxious. I took every symptom as a sign that something might be physically wrong with the pregnancy, and every negative interaction with my husband as a sign that the marriage might not work.

As my due date approached, I became even more afraid of labor and delivery, and I tried to learn all kinds of techniques for pain and anxiety reduction. I told people that I imagined giving birth and becoming a mother as a big waterfall looming in front of me. I couldn't see what was on the other side, and I didn't know anything about what would happen and what my life would be like afterward. But I knew it would be dramatic and possibly traumatic, and that I would never be the same again.

Then my due date came, and I had to be induced because my water broke but labor didn't start. Eventually it was more and more clear that I wasn't progressing, and I'd probably need a C-section. But I held out as long as possible, hoping to have a vaginal birth. When I finally had the C-section after thirty-two hours, I was completely exhausted and traumatized by the pain, fear, and uncertainty. I felt like a failure because my body hadn't done what I thought it should be able to do. I couldn't get pregnant on my own, and then I couldn't even give birth normally.

The baby and I had trouble with breast-feeding, and I hardly slept for two months, trying to work on it. The baby cried a lot and had trouble sleeping, probably because he wasn't getting enough calories. We went to a lactation consultant, had postpartum doulas, and went to the pediatrician frequently to weigh the baby and see if he was gaining more weight. I remember thinking that everyone I spoke to—nurses in the hospital, our pediatrician, lactation consultants, doulas—was contradicting each other. The more help I sought out, the more confused I felt.

Increasingly I felt despair, that I was incompetent as a mother and couldn't possibly take care of this baby. My body was more exhausted than I thought was possible, between not sleeping, recovering from major abdominal surgery, bleeding profusely for weeks, and expending so much energy trying to increase my milk production. I felt what-ever energy I had was leaking out with the milk. I sat and breast-fed for most of the day and night. My life was the couch and my nipples and the baby crying. I felt hopeless and helpless, and didn't know how I could go on.

Finally after two months, I started supplement-ing with formula. The baby instantly slept better with a full tummy, and I was relieved. But I still usually got up for every feeding at night, and my sleep-deprived mind became more and more des-perate. I would hear the baby crying even when he wasn't. Sometimes when I was walking down the hallway at three a.m. with the baby crying in my arms, I pictured myself throwing him against the wall. I was horrified. I had always loved children and thought of myself as a nurturing, mothering kind of person. I lost all faith in myself and didn't know who I was anymore. I wondered if I was going crazy, or if I was really a violent, destructive person rather than the gentle person I had thought I was. I told myself and other people that I couldn't take care of the baby, that I couldn't be a mother. I was afraid to leave the house with the baby. It was hard enough meeting his needs at home; out in the world it seemed almost impossible.

I started to get anxiety attacks as evening approached. I didn't know how I would take care of the baby—feed him, and especially get him to sleep. He was dependent on being held or nursed to fall asleep, and he stayed up way too late at night, reawakening frequently. I always felt like I was winging it, like I had no idea what to do and whether things would work out.

I looked at the baby when we were out in public and didn't feel connected to him. He looked nothing like me, which made me wonder how we were related if not genetically. I kept feeling like I wasn't a "real mom." Maybe it was just being so new at it, or the depression, or confusion about how to reconcile the fact that I was infertile and yet had produced a baby. I also felt like I wasn't a "real mother" because I needed so much more help with the baby than I thought I should need.

Eventually I became so depressed and anxious that it was hard for me to get out of bed in the morning. I lay in bed and thought about how my husband was mean, crazy, and didn't care about me. I felt trapped and hopeless. I could not imagine ever again feeling pleasure, peace, love, confidence, or joy. I couldn't remember ever feeling rested, relaxed, strong, or healthy.

Finally I decided I needed to get on antidepressants. I found a wonderful psychiatrist who helped me get past my intense fear of psychiatric medication and prescribed a low dose of sertraline (Zoloft). Soon I was able to function better, and I wasn't as debilitated as my depression and anxiety lifted significantly.

Then I hired a sleep consultant when the baby was six months old. The baby was awakening more and more frequently at night, had erratic naps, and was harder to soothe. I knew we needed to do sleep training, but I felt panicky whenever I thought about letting him cry himself to sleep. I thought my job as mother was to keep the baby from ever crying. But I was so desperate for sleep, and the baby had become inconsolable and unable to sleep for more than an hour at a time, so I was willing to try anything.

My husband volunteered to be in charge of sleep training. He knew I wouldn't be able to handle it, that I'd break down and pick up the baby. He read sleep training books over and over. He gave me earplugs and told me to stay in our bedroom with the door closed. The first night, the baby cried for less than an hour and then slept all night! It was like a miracle. I awoke in the morning, after the first full night's sleep I'd had, and felt ecstatic! My depression was completely gone. Knowing that I was off-duty at night from now on was so freeing. Being able to sleep all night was pure luxury, and I was so relieved and amazed to find out that our baby, who I thought was simply incapable of sleeping well, was actually a great sleeper. I realized that I hadn't kept up with the baby's development. I had still been treating him like a newborn who was completely dependent on adults. Actually, all he had needed was for us to teach him how to sleep independently. He had been sleep deprived and inconsolable at night because he wanted to sleep but didn't know how.

My husband and I went to marriage counseling at my insistence. I felt like I couldn't feel completely recovered as long as we hadn't healed the rift that had gotten so bad during my depression. We learned to express our feelings in a nonthreatening way and to really hear each other. We started to empathize with and understand each other, even though we are so different. Now we are more flexible with each other and can work out our conflicts peacefully. I now feel supported and loved, and I know that my husband is trying his best to make me happy. We are now both really enjoying parenting together.

In individual therapy I learned to stop blaming myself for my anxiety and PPD. I forgave myself for not living up to my high expectations for myself. I started to feel that I was living my life as a functional person, instead of just struggling to get through each day.

I've gone from just feeling anxious about being a mother, constantly worried about what to do and whether my baby was all right, to really enjoying motherhood. My son is eighteen months old now, and I have so much fun with him! He has taught me how to enjoy the moment and not think about the past or the future. He reaches for me and calls me "Mama," and now I feel like a mama, like his mama.

Remember: It's important to allow others to help you. You don't have to do everything on your own to be a good mother.

Exercise

There is plenty of data regarding the positive effects of exercise for body and mind. Although exercise isn't recommended as the sole treatment, it should be a part of every treatment plan. Exercise helps relieve depression with the population as a whole—even major depression. In one study (Babyak et al., 2000), participants doing only exercise for four months had the same improvement with less relapse than the group using sertraline (Zoloft) only or the group using both exercise and sertraline. Exercise elevates serotonin and dopamine in the brain (important mood-regulating chemicals) and releases endorphins ("happy" chemicals). Inflammation, regarded by many researchers as a major cause of depression, is lowered by moderate exercise, and that's one of the reasons why these researchers believe that exercise helps alleviate depression. What is considered "moderate" depends on your fitness level. However, while exercise can ease the physiological symptoms of depression, it should never replace therapy. Exercise along with the life skills learned in therapy can be a wonderful combination.

EXERCISE IN PREGNANCY

The American College of Obstetricians and Gynecologists recommends thirty minutes of moderate exercise on most days during pregnancy. One study of nondepressed pregnant women showed that the exercisers had less depressive symptoms in the first and second trimesters compared to those who did not exercise. Another study demonstrated that the effects of a single aerobic exercise session had more benefits for mood than the control group. There was a significant decrease in anxiety and depression for both pregnant and postpartum women. If you are experiencing panic, however, don't do too much heavy aerobic exercise even if the doctor has given you a go-ahead. Pushing yourself too much can make adrenaline surge through your system, making the panic worse. Also, lactic acid makes you sore from too much exercise, and lactic acid can also cause panic.

There is a particular exercise program that stands out from the others. It involves no equipment, it's nonimpact, and it's quick (a workout is five to seven minutes). Physiologists, biologists, and chemists who have studied this system have determined how it works, and the results of the research studies from the University of Utah explain why this program is superior compared to traditional exercise programs. The OBs to whom I have shown the program and the research are in agreement that pregnant women benefit from using it, and the OBs and other M.D.s who already endorse the system regularly prescribe it to their patients—pregnant and nonpregnant. Studies show that compared to the other exercise methods tested, with this system nine times more body fat is burned, six times more lean muscle is generated (compared to weight training), twenty-one times the fat is lost, and twelve and a half times the oxygen intake/respiratory capacity is increased. The research shows vastly and immediately improved flexibility and strength more than all other exercises tested. This system immediately generates a huge amount of oxygen in the cells, and there is extensive exercise to the diaphragm and vital organs, which increases circulation of the lymph and circulatory systems. With this system, oxygen is available to the body before the nerve centers determine there's a decrease, so you won't find yourself out of breath and panting. This phenomenon also keeps the heart rate low, among other benefits, so if you have a panic disorder, there's less of a worry that your adrenaline will shoot up and give you a panic attack. Health practitioners have noticed there is less soreness reported by their patients compared to traditional exercises, meaning that the lactic acid buildup is probably minimal. (Remember, lactic acid can cause anxiety and panic.) Feel free to visit www.znatrainer.com for more information, and check with your doctor before beginning any exercise program.

Just Do What You Can

Pregnancy can make it difficult to want to move your body, due to fatigue or discomfort. Add depression on top, and there's another layer of lack of motivation. Start from wherever you are, and do what you can to move your body—any way you do, consider it exercise. If you walk to the mailbox, that's great. If all you're able to do one day is move from the bedroom into the living room, then good for you. Get outside for some sunshine and air, even if it's just to walk half a block or one circle around your yard. In this society, the images of exercise are pretty narrow, like going to the gym, biking, or swimming. Expand your concept of exercise and feel great about yourself for whatever you're able to do each day, since it will depend on how you feel both physically and emotionally. If you are unable to leave your bed for physical or emotional reasons, www.znatrainer.com has a program you may be interested in. Check with your doctor before beginning any exercise program.

Exercise Warning

If you find that you are exercising compulsively and you're afraid that if you miss a day of exercise then you'll feel depressed or anxious, that's not normal. Or if you feel you need to be exercising for hours every day to keep your head on straight, that's a warning sign that your brain chemistry needs something else in addition to exercise. Many exercise addicts you meet are actually suffering from mood disorders, and they're trying to keep their brain chemistry normal by self-medicating with exercise. This is a never-ending treadmill (no pun intended). It's an unhealthy cycle (another pun—sorry). Seriously, you should be able to skip a day of exercise without feeling like you're going to "lose it."

YOGA

In 2005 research was done to study the effectiveness of yoga on pregnancy outcomes (Narendran et al.). The research wasn't specifically geared toward helping mood disorders in pregnancy, but the types of health benefits witnessed in the yoga group were significant and implied that yoga would most likely help with moods as well. One hundred and sixty-nine women were in the yoga group, and 166 women were in the control group (no yoga). Physical postures, breathing, and meditation were practiced for an hour each day from about eighteen weeks pregnant until delivery. The control group walked thirty minutes twice a day, which is standard advice given by OBs. For the "yoga moms" the birth weight of their babies was significantly higher, preterm labor was significantly lower, and complications such as intrauterine growth retardation and high blood pressure due to pregnancy were also significantly lower. An educated guess is that stress levels were also lower in these moms.

Folate

Folate (also known as folic acid) is an important key to prenatal nutrition, and it is also thought to help antidepressants work better and more quickly. A water-soluble B vitamin that's found naturally in food, including leafy greens (like spinach and turnip greens), legumes, and some fruits, it's similar to SAMe (refer to the SAMe section later in this chapter) in terms of how it helps metabolism. Depression is associated with low folate levels, and those with low folate levels tend not to respond well to antidepressants. Adding folate, however, can help the antidepressant work for them.

The body needs folate to make and maintain new cells, and this is especially important when rapid cell division and growth is occurring (such as during pregnancy and in infancy). Folate is necessary to make DNA and RNA, the building blocks of cells. In addition, folate helps prevent abnormal changes in DNA that may cause cancer. Everyone needs folate to make normal red blood cells and prevent anemia. Since 1998, food manufacturers in the United States have been required to add folic acid (the synthetic form of folate) to many foods, such as breads, pastas, cereals, grain products, and flours. These regulations were put in place to decrease the risk of neural tube birth defects in newborns. Since then, those in the United States, whether they know it or not, have been relying on the folic acid added to foods to receive this vitamin. Folic acid, while synthetic, is just as effective as folate, and it actually is absorbed more easily by the body.

It's recommended that men and women over age nineteen should take 400 micrograms (mcg) of folic acid every day. During pregnancy the Recommended Daily Allowance (RDA) is 600 mcg.

FOLATE IN PREGNANCY

Folate has been found to help with major depression, is safe in pregnancy, and helps to boost the effect of an antidepressant. Although there's no specific study of folate in pregnancy, women who plan to get pregnant are told to take folate daily to decrease birth defects. Taking enough folate before pregnancy and during pregnancy (and lactation) is crucial for the baby's development, and it protects the baby from a number of congenital malformations, including neural tube defects (malformations of the spine, brain, and skull). The risk of neural tube defects decreases considerably when folate is taken in addition to eating a healthful diet before and during the first month of pregnancy.

Again, the RDA for folate (or folic acid) during pregnancy is 600 micrograms, and most prenatal vitamins include this amount.

> Folate has been found to help with major depression, is safe in pregnancy, and helps to boost the effect of an antidepressant.

Homeopathy

Even though you can walk into any health-food store and see little bottles of homeopathic remedies for depression, anxiety, or other ailments, it's wise to keep walking. Don't try to treat yourself with these remedies. There are practitioners of homeopathy (some of whom are medical doctors or naturopathic doctors) who report positive results treating patients for depression and anxiety, but there is very little published data on the subject. To be officially certified as a practitioner, three or four years of training is required; however, there is very little regulation in this area. Although there is no scientific data yet supporting the safety or effectiveness of homeopathy in pregnancy, both are claimed by the field. Many women attribute their wellness in part to working with a skilled practitioner who provides remedies made just for them. If you wish to work with a homeopathic practitioner, a good source for finding a certified homeopath is the Council for Homeopathic Certification (CHC). As always, you will still want to interview the practitioner regarding his or her training and experience dealing with your particular health concerns.

Light Therapy

Since there are at least two types of therapy that fall into this category, I'm presenting each of them, because the methods used are quite different and they work differently in the brain.

PHOTOTHERAPY

Bright-light therapy (phototherapy) is very effective in treating Seasonal Affective Disorder (SAD), and it also helps to normalize sleeping patterns. A study in the *American Journal of Psychiatry* (2000) that focused on depressed new mothers found this type of therapy helpful. In phototherapy, you use a special light box in your house or in a professional's office. Your eyes are open, but you're not staring directly into the light. Depending on your specific needs, the professional prescribes phototherapy for you to do sometime during the day for a particular length of time and number of days per week. Usually the doctor will have you start for just a few minutes (maybe five) a day and work up from there. Some women with bipolar illness can have a manic response to bright-light therapy—just because this therapy employs light, and light is natural, doesn't mean that it's not a powerful treatment. Light boxes are easy to find these days since the public demand is so high, but the quality (and therefore, effectiveness) of these boxes do differ, so check with your health practitioner before purchasing one. Also, depending upon your condition, this therapy may or may not be appropriate for you. As always, please don't self-treat. If you've been given the go-ahead by your doctor, easy guidelines for purchasing a light box on your own can be found on www.cet.org.

PHOTOTHERAPY IN PREGNANCY

There are two studies supporting light box therapy in pregnancy, and at least one other clinical trial is currently underway. One bright-light study for depressed pregnant women showed that after three weeks of using light therapy for sixty minutes in the morning, depression scores improved by 49 percent. For the women who completed five weeks, their scores improved by 59 percent. Withdrawal of the light therapy caused most of the women to relapse. There are few negative side effects to light therapy when treating depression, but if you have bipolar disorder, your doctor may prescribe a different regimen

There are few negative side effects to light therapy when treating depression, but if you have bipolar disorder, your doctor may prescribe a different regimen for you since it can cause manic symptoms.

for you since it can cause manic symptoms. No matter what your diagnosis, please check with your medical doctor before using it. Typically, psychiatrists prescribe the use of a light box, but other medical doctors are learning about the benefits and coming on board with this treatment as well. There are light boxes that are more effective than others, and your doctor will recommend a good one. Or you can go to www.cet .org for the important facts to look for when purchasing a light box. On this site you can also access studies on bright-light therapy for pregnant women (the term you'll see is *antenatal*, meaning "during pregnancy").

BLOCKING BLUE LIGHT

Melatonin, called the sleep hormone because it makes you drowsy, reaches its maximum concentration during the night. Light causes the pineal gland, which makes melatonin, to reduce production of melatonin. If the schedule on which the pineal gland is producing melatonin is out of synch with the sleep schedule, sleep problems will result. In order to alleviate this, a treatment has been devised to increase melatonin by blocking light. Two recent studies have found that the suppression of melatonin by light depends on the color of the light, and that it's specifically the blue component that suppresses melatonin. This treatment involves glasses, developed by researchers from John Carroll University, that help the brain's natural melatonin continue to be produced by blocking more than 95 percent of blue light, even when you're awake. You wear the glasses for one to three hours before bed (you take them off to sleep). The glasses have demonstrated effectiveness with bipolar disorder in research studies (James Phelps, M.D., Corvallis Psychiatric Clinic), and additional trials are currently being performed.

BLOCKING BLUE LIGHT IN PREGNANCY

The results of an eight-week double-blind postpartum sleep study that I conducted indicate that there was a 96.7 percent chance that the improvement of the participants' sleep was not due to chance—in other words, it was the sleep glasses that enhanced the quality of the women's sleep. Unlike the postpartum study, a pregnancy study conducted concurrently was not double blind (there's no placebo—every woman was sent the "real" pair), so it is less scientific. However, during the eight weeks, the participants reported the same things as the postpartum participants with the "real" pair. Comments included, "I can go back to sleep if I need to get up during the night," "I fall asleep more easily," "I'm dreaming more," and "I don't toss and turn as much." You can find more information on these glasses by going to lowbluelights.com.

Omega-3 Fatty Acids

These essential fatty acids have been studied more than any of the other CAM treatments. Omega-3 fatty acids are comprised of eicosapentenoic (EPA) and docosahexanoic (DHA), both found in fish. Research shows that omega-3 creates significant treatment benefit in mood disorders, and in most studies, omega-3 fatty acids have been added to a regimen of antidepressant medications. Depression is ten times more common in countries where fish isn't eaten as much, and these findings led an expert panel of the American Psychiatric Association to conclude that EPA was a promising treatment for mood disorders.

OMEGA-3 IN PREGNANCY

Many research groups have found that pregnant women become depleted in omega-3 since the baby uses it for its nervous system development. With each subsequent pregnancy, mothers are further depleted. This may explain why postpartum mood disorders may become worse—even beginning earlier in pregnancy—with subsequent pregnancies. When a mother is deficient in omega-3, it increases her risk for depression. Hibbeln's 2002 study found that mothers who ate high amounts of seafood during pregnancy, and who had high levels of DHA in their milk postpartum, had lower levels of postpartum depression. (Note: If you're a vegetarian, please note that flaxseed has omega-3, but it doesn't provide EPA or DHA and has not been demonstrated to have a helpful effect on depression.)

Omega-3 fatty acids (referred to here as "omega-3s") have many positive benefits: benefiting your baby's retinal and brain function, reducing inflammation, improving cardiovascular health, treating high triglycerides, and possibly preventing dementia. Most importantly, however, research we now have on omega-3s show that these essential fatty acids may help treat and prevent depression in pregnancy and postpartum. Numerous studies have shown that higher amounts

> ## *Eating Fish during Pregnancy*
> *It's important to fully understand the FDA's (www.fda.gov) warnings about fish intake for pregnant women. It states that pregnant women should avoid four species of fish that have high mercury content: shark, swordfish, tilefish, and king mackerel. (Forgoing tilefish is not much of a sacrifice for most Americans.) Other fish should be limited to twelve ounces per week, which is still a good amount and a good source of omega-3 and protein. Many of the most popularly eaten fish are thought to be safe, such as salmon. For the fish with the most omega-3 fatty acids, opt for wild versus farmed fish.*

of omega-3s from seafood intake correlate to lower rates of depression in general, postpartum depression, bipolar disorder, and suicide. The human body does not produce omega-3 on its own, so it continually needs to input more. The most efficient source of the most important omega-3 fatty acids (EPA and DHA) is fatty cold-water fish, like salmon and tuna. Many pregnant women are afraid to eat fish due to contaminants such as mercury, and while that's unfortunate, it's okay because supplements are available. It's important, however, to choose a reputable, high-quality brand of supplement, since the refinement process for these better brands removes contaminants like mercury, and the oil is fresh, as opposed to the rancid oil used by many lesser brands. (If you find there is a "fishy" aftertaste to the supplement you are using, the oil is probably rancid.) Even with an omega-3 supplement, it's still good to eat fish, since fish is an important source of numerous other nutrients, including protein. Also, many of the known benefits associated with omega-3 fatty acids in pregnant women were derived from population studies that looked at fish intake.

SAMe

S-Adenosyl Methionine (SAMe), a molecule that occurs naturally and is important for metabolism, has been used in Europe for over twenty years, but it's been slower to gain popularity in the United States. Methionine, an essential amino acid that breaks down in the liver to produce SAMe, is necessary for the normal functioning of brain chemicals (neurotransmitters) that control mood, such as serotonin and dopamine. In healthy brains, amino acids produce enough SAMe, but this isn't true for those with depression. SAMe works best when it's taken in conjunction with folate and Vitamin B12. It can be used both instead of a standard antidepressant as well as in addition to an antidepressant, since it can help the antidepressant work better. It's often better tolerated and works faster than many prescribed antidepressants. For nonpregnant or nursing women, the typical dosage of SAMe is 400 milligrams taken three to four times a day. After a few weeks, you may be able to lower your dosage to 200 milligrams two times a day.

SAMe IN PREGNANCY

Studies in treating pregnant women with liver problems have demonstrated that SAMe helps both with liver disease and general liver functioning. Moms and babies did very well, reported the Agency for Healthcare Research and Quality (AHRQ, 2002). Many professionals agree that it's also safe to take while breast-feeding, and it has been used effectively as a treatment for postpartum depression. (There are other professionals who feel the safety of SAMe in pregnancy and breast-feeding has not been clearly established yet.) Studies show there are fewer side effects with SAMe than with the older tricyclic antidepressants. The only possible danger I know of with SAMe is that it may cause mania in someone with bipolar disorder, the same way a standard antidepressant can. Make sure to tell your doctor if you're taking SAMe.

St. John's Wort (Hypericum)

Herbs are powerful medicine and shouldn't be taken lightly. Remember that just because something is natural, that doesn't automatically make it safe. With that said, St. John's Wort is an extremely popular herb used in Europe as a first choice to treat depression over a standard antidepressant. The results of studies on St. John's Wort are extremely mixed, however. Some conclude that St. John's Wort is just as effective as standard antidepressants. There is research showing that this herb is only effective to treat mild to moderate depression, but there is also research showing that it can effectively treat severe depression. However, large studies in the United States failed to find benefit of St. John's Wort for major depression, making many professionals skeptical. It should never be taken with an SSRI antidepressant, hormone replacement therapy, or oral contraceptives because of negative interactions. St. John's Wort interferes with the effectiveness of the hormones in oral contraceptives, which can cause unwanted pregnancy. Always tell your doctor if you're using this herb.

ST. JOHN'S WORT IN PREGNANCY

The data regarding the safety of St. John's Wort in pregnancy and with breast-feeding is a bit confusing. In one study of thirty-three pregnant women treated with St. John's Wort, their newborns had increased colic, drowsiness, and lethargy as compared with infants born to depressed and nondepressed moms not taking the herb. St. John's Wort seems to be a good first choice for those who are not pregnant or nursing (it also lowers inflammation), but there isn't enough data regarding the safety of the herb for those who are pregnant or nursing. Although it's thought by most to probably be safe for breast-feeding, more study is needed to understand the long-term effects on children.

Key Points

- *As with any health provider, you will want to interview prospective CAM practitioners regarding their training and experience before signing on for treatment.*

- *Many traditional medical practitioners are embracing integrative medicine, a type of medicine that takes into account the whole person—body, mind, and soul.*

- *Due to its positive effects on body and mind, exercise should be a part of every treatment plan.*

Chapter 8

NUTRITION FOR BODY AND MIND

Feeding your brain the nutrients it needs can make the difference between suffering and not suffering with mood problems. Nutrition is powerful at controlling your mood, and it plays a vital role in your mental health and overall well-being during and after pregnancy—for that matter, throughout your lifetime. While it remains crucial to eat a healthy, well-balanced diet at all times, it's never more important than during pregnancy and breast-feeding. Furthermore, the dietary needs of pregnant and breast-feeding women are substantially different than the dietary needs of others. As you read through this chapter, please—especially if you tend to obsess—keep breathing and don't get overwhelmed. If you're pregnant, you've probably already received lists of dos and don'ts, which can feel burdensome. This chapter isn't meant to add to any feeling of pressure. To the contrary, I want to help you lighten up. It's here to help guide you so that you'll be in the best position to feel well—mentally and physically—throughout your pregnancy.

Food Groups and Preparation

As you already know, a well-balanced diet consists of eating from a mixture of different food groups. What you may not know is that rather than compartmentalizing food into categories like "dairy" and "meat," foods are more accurately evaluated by their content. For example, the "meat group" is really the "protein group." Foods found in this category can be anything from steak and tofu to peanut butter and beans—all of which are high in protein.

Two other important categories to consider while planning your meals and grocery lists are raw and organic foods. Raw food is important because the more food is cooked, the more of its nutrients are stripped away. Also, when food is cooked or heated, especially by barbecuing and frying, it creates microscopic bits of "burnt" matter in the food. Just like smoke, charcoal, or ash, these burnt microbes are toxic in our bodies. So to be on the safe side, whenever possible replace frying and barbecuing with boiling, steaming, and poaching. Organic food is also important because it will help you avoid adding more pollution to your body. This pollution includes pesticides, antibiotics, hormones, and food that has been genetically modified. You can buy organic veggies, meat, dairy products, and eggs in most regular grocery stores.

Eating Right for You

A large body of new research shows that each person has different nutrition needs. In other words, you may need to eat different things as compared to your neighbor in order to be balanced. There are three different nutritional body types: protein, carbohydrate, and mixed. A "protein type" needs to eat a low-carbohydrate, high-protein, high-fat diet. A "carbo-hydrate type" needs to eat about 60 percent carbohydrates, 25 percent protein, and 15 percent fat. To figure out where you belong, simply analyze how you feel after either a high-carbohydrate or a high-protein meal by answering the following questions:

Did you feel hungry even though you were full of food?

Did you crave sweets after you ate?

Did your energy level drop?

Did you become hyper, nervous, angry, irritable, or depressed?

After eating a high protein meal, a protein type will feel good—satisfied, and with no digestion, energy, blood sugar, or mood problems. A carbohydrate type will have some or all of these issues after eating a high protein meal. The reverse is true when the types eat a high carbohydrate meal.

Eating well should always be part of your regimen, but especially during and after pregnancy. Focus on not only eating right for your type but on eating foods that contain necessary vitamins and minerals. Additionally, in your first trimester you should aim to eat an extra 150 calories more per day than you normally would. In your last two trimesters, you'll need 350 calories more per day. Most doctors recommend that you gain between twenty-five and thirty pounds if you are a healthy weight at the time of conception.

New research shows that each person has different nutrition needs. You may need to eat different things as compared to your neighbor in order to be balanced.

My Favorite Nutritional System

There is a nutritional system that has most of what you need in pregnancy contained within it. It is the simplest and highest-quality nutritional system I know of for pregnant and new moms. Included among the benefits reported are a decrease in sugar cravings, more stable and positive moods, increased energy (the steady and upbeat kind, not the nervous kind), and a decrease in "brain fog." I'm purposely not mentioning the system's name here since it's important that you order only those products that are appropriate for you, depending on your situation. For instance, if you're preparing for pregnancy, you can use all of the products; but if you're already pregnant, only some of them will be appropriate for you to use. Feel free to contact me for more information through ClearSky-Inc.com.

Important Food Groups

Vitamin- and Mineral-Rich Calcium Foods

Calcium is necessary to keep your bones from becoming depleted and to help your baby's bones develop. You need about 1,000 milligrams of calcium per day when you are pregnant or breast-feeding, which is going to be about 400 milligrams more than you need when you aren't pregnant or breast-feeding.

Some examples of serving sizes for calcium-rich foods are listed here:

- *Yogurt: 8 ounces. Flavored yogurts contain a lot of sugar, so opt for a plain, low-fat yogurt. You'll*

> *also want to avoid sugar-free yogurts that contain harmful artificial sweeteners. You can sweeten plain yogurt with fresh fruit, honey, or granola.*

- *Mozzarella cheese: 1.5 ounces. Cheeses that are white in color are healthier than cheeses that are yellow/orange. Not only do they not have dye in them, but they contain less harmful fat.*

- *Salmon: 3 ounces. Be sure that any seafood you eat is guaranteed to be pollutant-free. Try canned or fresh salmon (wild salmon is better than farm raised).*

- *Spinach: 2 cups. Substitute spinach for lettuce on a sandwich whenever possible and add it to a salad. Fresh raw spinach has substantially more nutrition than spinach that has been baked or boiled.*

PROTEIN FOODS

Protein intake is crucial for your energy and the baby's full development. You'll need a minimum of 60 grams per day (more if you are a "protein type" or if you are pregnant with more than one baby). As far as postpartum depression is concerned, eating protein increases the amount of tyrosine in your brain, which, in turn, increases dopamine. Dopamine is a chemical that elevates your mood and enhances your energy and alertness. It can feel daunting to eat the amount of protein required, so protein shakes can be wonderful, assuming they have the right protein and are of the purest quality (refer to the system I mention earlier in the chapter, for instance). Nibbling high-quality protein throughout the day will help your blood sugar remain more stable and your moods more even.

Some examples of serving sizes for protein-rich foods are listed here:

- *Poultry: 3 ounces. Try boiling a skinless chicken, rather than barbecuing or frying.*

- *Salmon: 3 ounces. Be sure that any seafood you eat is guaranteed to be pollutant-free. Try canned or fresh wild salmon.*

- *Cottage cheese: 1 cup. If you have a hard time eating cottage cheese, try it with fresh fruit or sweetened with honey and cinnamon. You can also substitute it for yogurt in a fruit smoothie.*

- *Peanut butter: 2 tablespoons. A great way to have peanut butter is spread inside celery stalks.*

- *Eggs: 1 egg. Try a hard-boiled egg to avoid the traditional scrambled or fried egg that has been cooked in oil or butter. Be sure to get organic, omega-3 eggs.*

- *Swiss cheese: 3 ounces. Again, try to stick to white-colored cheeses.*

IRON-RICH FOODS

Try to eat between 22 and 27 milligrams of iron daily. A lack of iron in your diet can cause fatigue, which doesn't help depression. Other risks of iron deficiency in pregnancy include premature delivery and low birth weight.

Some examples of serving sizes for iron-rich foods are listed here:

- *Beans: 1 cup. Try adding kidney beans to a salad or cooking a ten-bean soup.*

- *Spinach: 2 cups. Once again, substitute spinach for lettuce on a sandwich whenever you can, and add a few spinach leaves to your salad.*

- *Beef: 3 ounces. Eat organic beef, and avoid barbecuing and frying.*

- *Turkey: 3.5 ounces. As with beef, eat organic and avoid barbecuing and frying.*

FRUITS AND VEGETABLES

You already know the importance of eating fruits and vegetables. Aim for five to seven servings of fruits and vegetables per day while you are pregnant or breast-feeding, and try to eat at least one serving of a fruit or vegetable high in vitamins A and C per day. For example, you need between 40 and 60 grams of vitamin C per day during and immediately after pregnancy. The nutritional system referred to earlier in the chapter has delicious products that take care of all your fruit and vegetable needs.

Some examples of serving sizes for various fruits and vegetables, as well as their vitamin content, are listed here:

- *Spinach: 2 cups (vitamin A)*

- *Chili pepper: 2 tablespoons (vitamins A and C)*

- *Tomato: 2 medium-size tomatoes (vitamins A and C)*

- *Vegetable juice cocktail: 6 ounces (vitamin A)*

- *Raw green onion: ½ cup (181.4 grams) (vitamin A)*

- *Apricot: 3 apricots (vitamin A)*

- *Papaya: ½ of a medium-size papaya (vitamin A)*

- *Mango or cantaloupe: ¼ of a medium-size mango or cantaloupe (vitamins A and C)*

- *Citrus juice: 6 ounces (vitamin C)*

- *Orange or lemon: 1 medium size orange or lemon (vitamin C)*

- *Grapefruit: ½ medium-size grapefruit (vitamin C)*

- *Tangerine: 2 medium tangerines (vitamin C)*

- *Kiwi/mango: 1 medium-size kiwi or mango (vitamin C)*

- *Strawberries: ½ cup (vitamin C)*

- *Broccoli: ½ cup (vitamin C)*

- *Brussel sprouts: ½ cup (vitamin C)*

- *Cauliflower: ½ cup (vitamin C)*

- *Cabbage: 1 cup (vitamin C)*

- *Red or green pepper: ½ cup (vitamins A and C)*

VITAMIN B-, IRON-, AND FIBER-RICH BREADS AND CEREALS

In general, carbohydrates should make up 45 to 60 percent of your diet—six to eleven servings—unless you are a "carbohydrate type," in which case carbohydrates can surely make up at least 60 percent of your diet. Regardless of your nutrition type, try to choose carbohydrates that are low on the glycemic index. *Glycemic* refers to glucose, which is sugar. The body turns carbohydrates into sugar, so, by choosing carbohydrates that are low on the glycemic index, you are essentially cutting down on your sugar intake. Carbohydrates that are low on the glycemic index include beans, lentils, cashews, and rice (brown rice is more nutritious than white). Carbohydrates to avoid include rice cakes, white bread, cornflakes, and baked potatoes. A good general rule to abide by is that the less processed the carbohydrate is, the better for you it will be (such as the difference between rice and rice cakes noted here).

Some examples of serving sizes for various forms of carbohydrates are listed here:

- *Tortilla: 1 tortilla. Try both corn and flour tortillas.*

- *Rice: ½ cup. Brown rice has more nutritional value because it hasn't been bleached. Opt for boiled or steamed rice rather than fried.*

- *Pasta: ½ cup. Steer clear of fatty Alfredo sauce and tomato sauce, which exacerbates heartburn. Try pesto sauce or garnish pasta with olive oil, herbs, chopped raw vegetables, and mozzarella cheese.*

- *Cereal: ¾ cup. Many cereals contain omega-3s and other nutrients that are important during and after pregnancy. Avoid sugary cereals, and try almond milk or yogurt with your cereal instead of cow's milk.*

- *Oatmeal: ½ cup. Instant oatmeal should be avoided as it is less nutritious than the old-fashioned oats and often comes in sugary flavors. Buy whole oats and sweeten with almond milk, raisins, fresh fruit, or sulfur-free dried fruit.*

- *Crackers: 1 ounce. Swiss or pepper jack cheese and crackers make for a delicious and nutritious snack.*

Typically, carbohydrate-type foods are where you are going to get your fiber as well. Some examples of serving sizes for various forms of fiber are listed here:

- *Banana: 1 (whole). Remember to buy organic.*

- *Apple (with skin): 1 medium apple. Buy organic. Also try with peanut butter or slices of white cheese.*

- *Orange juice: 8 fluid ounces. Also great for vitamin C.*

- *Beans: ½ cup. Again, try on a salad or in soup.*

- *Split pea soup: 1 cup. Great with crackers and white cheese.*

- *Flaxseed, ground: 1 tablespoon. Also a great*

*source of omega-3s, although not the kind that
helps depression.*

OTHER VITAMIN B (FOLATE/FOLIC ACID) FOODS

Vitamin B, also known as folate and folic acid, reduces your baby's risk of neural tube, brain, and spinal abnormalities. A deficiency in vitamin B increases the risk of premature delivery, low birth weight, and overall poor fetal growth. Studies also have shown that 15 to 38 percent of adults with depressive disorders have low levels of vitamin B. Additionally, raising folate levels in people suffering from depression leads to less fatigue and more mental clarity. Thiamine, or vitamin B1, has also been proven to improve one's mood. Your prenatal vitamin should have folic acid as one of the ingredients, but it's a good idea to also eat foods that contain folate.

Many sources of vitamin B have been listed earlier in this chapter, but since you need between 600 and 1,000 micrograms (1 milligram equals 1,000 micrograms) during and after pregnancy, I've listed more sources for you here:

- *Beef liver: 3 ounces. Remember to buy organic and avoid barbecuing.*

- *Spinach: 1 cup. Again, fresh spinach is great on a sandwich or in a salad.*

- *Great northern beans: ½ cup. Beans are also great on a salad or in a soup.*

- *Asparagus: 4 spears. Lightly steam asparagus, and you can serve with rice, salmon, garlic, and onion for a great meal.*

- *Oranges: 1 small orange. Buy organic!*

Fluids and Hydration

Taking in the necessary fluids during pregnancy and breast-feeding is much easier to do than some of the other elements of your "baby diet." While some controversy exists about the old adage of drinking eight glasses of water per day, the bottom line is to stay well hydrated. Water is not only necessary for your physical health, but also for your mental health. Dehydration can cause anxiety, so don't wait until you get thirsty. Bring some filtered room-temperature or slightly chilled water wherever you go and sip on it all day. Of course, fruit juice, vegetable cocktail, and decaffeinated herbal teas can also be on your menu. What shouldn't be on your menu is soda, coffee, and alcohol. Not only are they toxic for your body and for your baby's body, these drinks will dehydrate you, so you need to drink much more water to make up for this.

If you plan to breast-feed, it's a good idea to drink a large glass of water right before you feed your baby. Drinking the water before you nurse will ensure you don't forget to do it afterward, and you'll run less of a risk of feeling fatigue and anxiety—two side effects of dehydration. Staying hydrated will, therefore, help you stay upbeat and energetic, and help prevent mood problems in pregnancy and postpartum.

Fats

Eating the right amount and type of fats is critical to a healthy pregnancy and recovery, including minimizing your risk for prenatal and postpartum depression. Fats occur naturally in many of the foods you already eat, such as: butter, oils, salad dressings, olives, and avocados. When it comes to helping prevent depression, there is one particular type of fat you need to pay special attention to: omega-3s. Omega-3s were discussed in depth in chapter 7, but since this is the nutrition chapter, I'll mention these wonderful fats here as well.

Omega-3 fats have many positive benefits: improving retinal and brain function, reducing inflammation, controlling muscle contractions, lowering blood pressure and body temperature, improving memory, and regulating blood clotting, nerve transmission, kidney function, and allergic responses. Most importantly, however, research we now have on omega-3s indicates that these essential fatty acids help treat and prevent depression in pregnancy and postpartum. Numerous studies have shown that high amounts of omega-3s correlate to lower rates of depression in general, postpartum depression, bipolar disorder, and suicide.

> Numerous studies have shown that high amounts of omega-3s correlate to lower rates of depression in general, postpartum depression, bipolar disorder, and suicide.

The human body does not produce omega-3 on its own, so it continually needs to input more. It's practically impossible to consume the necessary amount of omega-3 for proper brain and body functioning just by eating food. Without supplementing with omega-3 fish oil capsules, the human body becomes deficient, especially during pregnancy and breast-feeding. If your prenatal vitamin doesn't have at least 3,000 milligrams of omega-3, you might want to use an omega-3 supplement in addition to the prenatal vitamin.

Omega-6, also very important, has a different story. A good ratio of omega-6 to omega-3 is 2:1. In Western diets today, the ratio is more like 16:1: deficient in omega-3 and overloaded with omega-6. Excessive amounts of omega-6 polyunsaturated fatty acids (PUFA) and a very high omega-6/omega-3 ratio promote cardiovascular disease, cancer, and inflammatory and autoimmune diseases. The lower the ratio becomes (the more omega-3 balances the omega-6), the healthier the person becomes in these areas. One of the main problems in the era of fast and processed foods is that the amount of omega-6 fatty acids in people's diets has grown to the point that many people have too much in their system, so the ratio is out of whack. Omega-6 is found in french fry oil (vegetable, corn, and safflower oils) and many other modern dishes. On the other hand, omega-3s, polyunsaturated fats typically found in plants and seafood, are consumed less and less each year. Pregnant and breast-feeding women are at high risk for being low in omega-3s because the baby takes it from the mother's system for its nervous system development. Therefore, it is particularly important to eat EPA (eicosapentenoic) and DHA (docosahexanoic), the long-chain form of omega-3s found in fish oil. (Be aware that flaxseed, a popular source of omega-3s, contains ALA (alpha-linolenic acid), not DHA or EPA. In other words, flaxseed, while nutritious and helpful with things like breast milk production, does not help prevent depression as far as we know.

Because each pregnancy a woman experiences contributes to the depletion of her "maternal reserves" of omega-3s and other nutrients, it becomes more and more important with each pregnancy to eat enough omega-3s. This continued depletion puts women with multiple pregnancies at higher risk of developing prenatal as well as postpartum depression. Let your doctor know if you are supplementing your diet with fish oil.

INFLAMMATION

To expound on the dangers of eating too many omega-6s, an excess is also responsible for increasing inflammation in your body. Inflammation is yet another factor many experts believe contributes to postpartum depression. While your body will naturally become inflamed in the months before delivery, omega-6s can elevate that healthy level of inflammation and, in turn, lead to preterm birth. Depression in pregnancy also increases your chances of delivering the baby too early. Many experts believe that excess inflammation is a significant factor in this statistic.

As you've begun to see, omega-6s and omega-3s function together. While too many omega-6s can elevate your chances of becoming depressed, too few omega-3s can also lead to becoming overly inflamed. Numerous studies have confirmed this relationship. Additionally, you can fight inflammation by increasing your antioxidants and keeping your blood sugar down (eating the right carbohydrates and limiting sugars and processed foods).

Supplements

Before I discuss prenatal or postpartum vitamins or supplements, understand that the body does not easily digest most of these pills, and therefore it doesn't gain full nutritional benefit from them. The benefit you reap depends largely on the quality of your vitamins. If you can find a prenatal vitamin that is powdered and put in capsules, that's ideal, since

If you can find a prenatal vitamin that is powdered and put in capsules, that's ideal, since the fine powder can be broken down and absorbed by your body more easily than a hard pill.

the fine powder can be broken down and absorbed by your body more easily than a hard pill (which often stays whole in your digestive tract).

I hear far too many pregnant women say, "I'm taking a prenatal multivitamin, so I don't need to be that careful about what I eat." This is flawed logic. Although I'm a firm believer in taking excellent vitamins and mineral supplements, you still need to eat according to the suggestions and servings explored in this chapter for the maximum health of your body.

If your doctor prescribes a prenatal vitamin that includes amounts of nutrients other than what I suggest here, follow your doctor's advice. Your prenatal multivitamin should probably include:

4,000–5,000 units of vitamin A
0.4–1.0 milligram of vitamin B (folic acid)
400 units of vitamin D (to include vitamin D3)
200–300 milligrams of calcium
70–200 milligrams of vitamin C
1.5 milligrams of thiamine
1.6 milligrams of riboflavin
2.6 milligrams of pyridoxine
17 milligrams of niacinamide
2.2 milligrams of vitamin B12
10 milligrams of vitamin E

15 milligrams of zinc
30 milligrams of iron
200 micrograms of selenium

If you're pregnant with or breast-feeding twins, your nutritional needs are a little different. Here is a basic list of essential nutrients you'll need:

4,000 calories
145 grams of protein
5,000+ units of vitamin A
100 milligrams of vitamin C
600 units of vitamin D
12 milligrams of vitamin E
2 milligrams of thiamine
2 milligrams of riboflavin
20 milligrams of niacin
3.2 milligrams of pyridoxine
1.25 milligrams of folic acid
5 micrograms of vitamin B12
1,600 milligrams of calcium
100 milligrams of iron
600 milligrams of magnesium
1,600 milligrams of phosphorous
3,250 milligrams of potassium
150 micrograms of iodine
25 milligrams of zinc

Vegetarian Diet While Pregnant

Protein! Protein! Protein! If you haven't tried protein bars, powders, shakes, high-protein meal replacement drinks (not to be used as a replacement but as a supplement during pregnancy and breast-feeding), or high-protein vegetarian meat substitutes, definitely consider adding these to your daily regimen. Because most crucial omega-3s are found in fish oil, consider making an exception for an omega-3 supplement. Lack of protein and deficiency in omega-3s can contribute to depression in pregnancy and postpartum, so it is crucial that you monitor your intake of these closely.

Key Points

- *Nutrition plays a vital role in mental health and well-being before, during, and after pregnancy.*

- *Nutritional needs vary from person to person, so it is important to know which nutritional "body type" you fall into, and eat accordingly.*

- *Prenatal vitamins alone will not satisfy all of your nutritional needs—you also need to eat right.*

- *Your prenatal vitamin will probably not have the optimal amount of omega-3 fish oil—you may need to eat more fish with omega-3, take an omega-3 supplement, or both.*

Chapter 9

YOUR RISK FOR POSTPARTUM DEPRESSION DURING AND AFTER DELIVERY

There are a number of factors that can make you high risk for postpartum depression or another postpartum mood or anxiety disorder. If you're reading this book, chances are you've experienced a mood or anxiety disorder, which automatically puts you at greater risk than others who haven't. This chapter discusses the main risk factors for a postpartum episode, and then, most importantly, outlines the basics to help avoid it. There's much you can do to minimize your risk, and I'm all in favor of prevention.

Laura's Story

I suffered, and recovered from, what I believe to be a very acute case of postpartum depression (PPD) even though I had an incredible pregnancy. I felt so

203

full of love and joy, and called my growing belly the best accessory ever. The first nine weeks after I gave birth were like a fairy tale. I was so happy and excited about our future. One day, out of the blue, my world came crashing down, with deep depression, intense anxiety, insomnia, despair, and OCD thoughts such as being afraid I would hurt my child. I was desperate for an end to the pain I was feeling, and any small amount of strength I had left in me at the end of the day after taking care of my son I dedicated to healing myself. I researched; I read; I called specialists. I did so much research that within weeks I had an arsenal of help—Dr. Bennett, one of the world's leading PPD doctors/therapists, a competent psychiatrist, antidepressant medication, an energy healer, and a great nutrition program. I did everything I could to get better. Every day I forced myself to get up and care for my son, hoping that each day would get better and that I would once again feel that love for my life and my son again. I felt so bad that I couldn't even muster up emotion for him besides doom.

Within three months, I was feeling much more like myself: I got my life back, regaining my joy about the future with my son, who I call my "Christmas morning" because every day I wake up with excitement and marvel at what new things he will be up to. I have weaned off the antidepressants completely and have felt great for over a year. As hard as PPD was to endure, I am a stronger person for it. I am more compassionate and take much better care of myself than I ever have.

My husband and I have thought long and hard about having another child, and while we have very normal fears, we are positive that it's what we want. The decision was fairly easy except for one thing—statistics say I will most likely develop PPD again. Most days I say, "No problem! I have my team! I have my tools!" Other days I feel doom and want to run in the other direction. I feel like my emotions are in a pinball machine! Arsenal or not, I am not looking forward to the possibility of feeling that pain again, even for a week, even for a day. But in my heart I know that being a mother to another child and watching my children grow up together far outweighs the fear or reality of another PPD episode.

My husband and I have been trying to conceive. We actually got pregnant right away but unfortunately had a very early miscarriage. The night that I found out I was pregnant, I felt extremely anxious and could hardly sleep fearing that not only would I suffer from PPD again, but maybe this time depression during pregnancy. My "what ifs" were in full motion. Luckily, I woke up the next morning feeling great. I was confident and knew I could handle whatever was thrown my way. Since the miscarriage, we have continued to try to conceive while I wean our twenty-month-old son. My hormones are again fluctuating because of weaning, and like many women, I am feeling depressed as a result. My "what ifs" keep popping up again, but I am working through it. What I do know is that my "what ifs" never come true! The answer is the same as before: I will be okay. I will be better than okay! I am an amazing mother and always say that there are two things that I know to be true—my love for my child and my ability to be the mother I always dreamed of being. Someone said to me the other day that if you are afraid you won't be able to love your second child as much as the first, not to worry. When you have your second child, your heart doesn't split in two, one side for each child—you grow a whole new heart. I like to think that if you have a second battle with PPD and once again win that battle, your spirit, wisdom, and strength doubles.

Remember: Some degree of worry is normal when you get pregnant again after a postpartum depression. But you've already got your team assembled and with proper help, you can have an emotionally healthy pregnancy

Frequently Asked Questions

SHOULD I WEAN OFF THE MEDICATION BEFORE I DELIVER? IF SO, WHEN?

Some well-meaning psychiatrists suggest weaning off antidepressants in the last month before delivery to help minimize the chances of the baby going through any withdrawal from the medication. However, most researchers and practitioners specializing in this field do not suggest this, since the mother will need the medication the very most at the time of delivery. For some women the precipitous drop in the reproductive hormones at birth may trigger postpartum depression, so it makes no sense to wean at the very moment that your brain chemistry needs the boost. The temporary and minimal side effects the baby may experience don't compare to the full-blown postpartum disorder that the woman may be thrust into if she eliminates the medication from her system at such a vulnerable time.

IF I WEAN OFF THE MEDICATION BEFORE DELIVERY, WHEN SHOULD I GET BACK ON IT AFTER THE BABY IS BORN? WHAT ARE THE WARNING SIGNS OF POSTPARTUM DEPRESSION?

Depending on your situation, you may want to pop that baby and pop that first dose right there on the delivery table. Remember that it can take a couple of weeks to start feeling the effects of the medication, and that's precious time you don't want to waste feeling miserable. Or some women do a "wait and see" and just look out for warning signs. If you have everything else in place—good nighttime sleep, excellent nutrition, breaks to nurture yourself, emotional and physical support—you can see if you still need medication. If so, you can always start taking it then. You can even have the prescription filled in advance just in case.

The warning signs and symptoms of postpartum depression are listed here, followed by the symptoms of other mood disorders. These lists were taken from my Web site, http:// ClearSky-Inc.com.

Postpartum depression affects about 15 percent of new mothers and may begin anytime during the first year postpartum. It is characterized by symptoms that include:

- *Anxiety*

- *Lack of energy*

- *Sleeping problems*

- *Confusion*

- *Frequent crying*

- *Low self-esteem*

- *Guilt feelings*

- *Appetite problems*

- *Irritability or anger*

- *Overwhelmed feelings*

- *Forgetfulness*

- *Decreased sex drive*

- *Mood swings*

- *Hopelessness*

Postpartum panic disorder is experienced by about 10 percent of new moms and may include:

- *Panic attacks*

- *Heart palpitations*

- *Chest pains*

- *Dizziness*

- *Nausea*

- *Hot or cold flashes*

- *Shaking*

- *Fear of losing control or going crazy*

- *Numbness or tingling*

Postpartum obsessive compulsive disorder is experienced by around 3 to 5 percent of mothers and often includes:

- *Obsessive and intrusive thoughts (sometimes including thoughts of hurting the baby)*

- *Avoidance of the baby*

- *Depression*

- *Anxiety*

- *Repetitive behaviors like counting (number of diapers in the bag, etc.)*

- *Checking (locking doors, baby's breathing, etc.) and cleaning*

Postpartum bipolar disorder (for which there aren't yet any statistics regarding prevalence) is characterized by:

- *Mania*

- *Rapid and severe mood swings*

- *Depression*

Postpartum psychosis, experienced by approximately 0.2 percent of mothers, is always a medical emergency. Symptoms include:

- *Extreme agitation*

- *Severe and rapid mood swings*

- *Incoherent statements*

- *Hallucinations*

- *Losing touch with reality*

Postpartum posttraumatic stress disorder affects between 1 and 6 percent of new moms with symptoms including:

- *Recurrent nightmares*

- *Extreme anxiety*

- *Reliving past traumatic events (sexual, physical, emotional, childbirth)*

AM I HIGH RISK FOR POSTPARTUM DEPRESSION?

If you've experienced postpartum depression in the past or if you've been depressed in pregnancy, the short answer is yes. If you've never been pregnant but you've had depression before, you're also high risk. However, high risk doesn't mean you'll definitely develop it (or develop it again). It just means you should prepare a plan of action just in case. Most of the plan discussed later in this chapter has nothing to do with medication. Rather, it's comprised of healthy steps that every woman and couple should have in place before delivery for two reasons: One, no woman is immune to postpartum depression, even if she has no history of depression. Two, most of the plan of action is healthy for every family.

High risk doesn't mean you'll definitely develop postpartum depression (or develop it again). It just means you should prepare a plan of action just in case.

Whether you're high risk also depends on what factors were in play during the previous depressions. For instance, if most of your depression was due to feeling isolated because you just moved to another location, that factor probably won't be present this time around, and you may not experience depression. But, generally speaking, if you have a personal or family history of depression, you're high risk for postpartum depression. The risk is higher still if you've had a postpartum depression before—around 80 percent. You're also very high risk if you've been depressed in pregnancy—especially in the third trimester. Other predictors are if you've had severe premenstrual syndrome (PMS) or premenstrual dysphoric disorder (PMDD), or if you've reacted with negative moods to a birth control pill. These are all situations when hormonal shifts have been present. If you've reacted in the past during these times, take this as a heads-up for depression after the delivery.

This is also true for the other mood disorders. For instance, if you have bipolar disorder or have reacted with a bipolar episode after a previous delivery, you're high risk now for another bipolar episode or even postpartum psychosis. If you've had a previous postpartum psychosis, you're at an extremely high risk, and you will probably want to immediately start antipsychotic medications upon delivery. If you've had panic attacks before, you're high risk for postpartum anxiety and panic, and if you have obsessive-compulsive disorder (OCD), you're high risk for worsening symptoms. With any trauma in your past that still haunts you, or possible scary experiences occurring in the upcoming delivery, it will put you at higher risk for postpartum posttraumatic stress disorder (PTSD).

Renee's Story

As I sit here tonight, when asked to recount my experience with this thing called postpartum depression, I am both happy and fearful. People may think I sound a little dramatic, but this experience has brought me to places I never knew existed. It has changed me forever and is something that I still think about and deal with daily.

I grew up somewhat misguided and lost as a teenager. Never the popular girl, I soon found my way after meeting my husband at nineteen. Something about getting married, growing up, and knowing him made me want to pursue more in life. And so I did. I went to school, became a nurse, and focused on my career. I felt powerful and in control of my life, more than I ever had. I was extremely independent and became very confident, knowing that if I wanted it, I could make it happen. It seemed like the world was at my feet.

I had always talked about having kids from the time we got married, but my husband wasn't ready. Finally, after about seven years of marriage, we started trying. By this time, I was of the attitude that I could take it or leave it. I was semi-content with my freedom, and part of me thought I could end up never having children. Two years later I was pregnant for the first time at thirty years old.

That morning after seeing that "pregnant" sign, I was immediately enveloped in a feeling of terror and shock—it was an immediate feeling of "oh my God, this thing is in me" and a deep realization that I could not escape this, no matter what. I was pregnant, and there was no turning back. Panic.

The pregnancy was filled with lots of worries, aches and pains, and strange things that I thought were signs that something was drastically wrong with my body or the baby. Now I know that there was nothing drastically wrong at all. Toward the third trimester I began to experience feelings of dizziness, fatigue, and weakness in my arms and legs. I even blacked out at a restaurant once. My midwife thought it was hypoglycemia. After a while I had a strong suspicion it was some sort of anxiety.

I had a wonderful birth, during which I was able to relax and focus all that energy into accomplishing a task—and I was successful, birthing an eight pound, thirteen ounce girl. It soon turned ugly, as after delivery I developed a life-threatening hematoma and went into shock. I lost a tremendous amount of blood that night as my husband, mother, and sisters looked on. I was sent home from the hospital two days later pale as a ghost, in pain, and ordered to be on bed rest for one week. The night I got home I had a massive panic attack. The baby was sleeping, and my mom told me to go to bed and get some sleep. I couldn't. There was too much going on in my mind. I did not want to be in another room away from my baby. I was terrified. It was so scary. Try to convince your mind that this is just another night and to go to sleep? What? I just brought home a baby who is mine, and they want me to actually sleep? I told my mom and husband that I thought I needed to go back to the hospital. My blood pressure was elevated, and I sat there across from my mom and husband shaking my head and telling them that there was something wrong with me. I felt so terrified. It was a feeling of life and death.

Over the next couple months I was still in a great deal of pain, so I couldn't stand for very long. I stayed in my bedroom with my baby, breast-feeding her, changing her, and sleeping with her there. I felt down, terrified that I would never be able to be a "proper mother" to my child and a wife to my husband. Six to eight weeks later I stopped bleeding, and the pain suddenly went away. My spirits lifted, and I felt on top of the world. I gushed about being a mother and how I loved it so, and I think I even remember saying I was meant to be a mother.

When my daughter turned about six or seven months old, right after I started her on solid food, I suddenly started feeling terrible. I felt like I needed to go outside and just run and run and run to burn off all the "electricity" or nervous energy I had. This kept up, and soon I dreaded waking up in the morning. I didn't want to get up and take care of my baby, but I did anyway. This was accompanied by feelings of total surrealism. I would drive down the street, and it felt like I was in a snow globe, if you can imagine. I couldn't grasp any glimmer of hope, not even looking at my daughter (my lowest point). I knew I loved her dearly, and that is what was so, so depressing and baffling and upsetting. Over the next six months I researched and sought help from many people for what I was experiencing, what I learned was called postpartum depression. I never took antidepressants, but I was prescribed them and encouraged to take them. I did take an occasional antianxiety drug during the worst time in the beginning to help me sleep, though. Those worked well. I was breast-feeding and was always ultra aware of effects on my sweet girl at the expense of myself.

It has been such a long and desperately hard road. I felt I was about 70 to 80 percent recovered when, about five months later, I learned I was pregnant again. My daughter was one year old. I was immediately happy, and then plunged into massive panic and fear, thinking what have I done? This was a very low time in my life, and I thought I could not do this for an entire pregnancy—no way! I struggled through the fatigue and nausea, and toward the end of the first trimester things started *going smoothly. I felt my first 100 percent day, and I began to enjoy my girl much more and feel like a real mom. I remember feeling that all those thoughts with PPD were not real. They are and were not me. They are not the real me.*

Today I am almost twenty-five weeks pregnant, and for the most part I've been doing well. I just recently over the last week or so have been feeling some old familiar feelings of anxiety, negative unwanted thoughts, and irritability with my husband and others. I always want to try and figure it out. Why am I feeling this now? Is it because I am under too much stress? What can I do to lessen that? Is it because I'm not exercising or drinking enough water? Too much sugar? Hormone surge? There are a million things I can blame it on, but the truth is I cannot and will not understand it. The most frustrating part is that I cannot predict it or stop and start my moods. I must work through it like before and try to employ all the routines and regimens that helped me last time. The one thing that I find helps me is to be around other people. It makes me feel normal again. One last and important note is to be thankful for the good moments, even if they only last a second. Stop immediately and say to yourself how wonderful this is, because it is. The truth is, my life is wonderful, and I have been blessed beyond belief. My experience of having kids has been the best of times and the worst of times. I look at it sometimes as this rite of passage, a challenge that is so difficult to the point where I want to give up, but I know in

> my soul that in the end it is going to be one of the
> most rewarding and cherished moments of my life.
> I hope I live to be an old woman, looking back and
> crying in joy and thanksgiving for my children and
> the struggle and the triumph.
>
> **Remember:** Depression and anxiety can begin
> months after the baby is born. But keep your per-
> spective. With proper help, the depressed and anx-
> ious times will eventually pass.

CAN I BREAST-FEED WHILE TAKING MY MEDICATION?

With very few exceptions (like lithium), if you can take it in
pregnancy, you can take it while breast-feeding. You don't
need to choose between taking a medication for your mental
health and breast-feeding your baby (or pumping your milk
into bottles).

If you're really concerned, there is a way to lower the
amount of medication your baby ingests. The literature doesn't
show any need for doing the following, and the huge effort
that pumping milk entails makes it undesirable. But because
some of my clients over the years have psychologically felt
better using this option, I'm mentioning it: You can "pump and
dump" the feeding right after the medication peaks in your
system (the number of hours differs for each medication). So
a bottle of formula or stored breast milk would be used for
that feeding in place of the just-pumped milk. Again, I'm not
advocating this practice since it's not needed and drains your
precious energy (and precious milk) and wastes it. But just in
case this offers you an in-between option that suits you, feel
free to use it.

If you feel you must choose between breast-feeding and taking an antidepressant, please try not to agonize over the decision. If you truly need the medication to feel well, the choice is a slam dunk. A calm, happy mother is more important to a child's healthy development than breast milk. The most important gift to your baby is a happy, healthy mother. Ignore whatever pressure may be around you regarding the need to breast-feed, and be assured that you're doing what's best for your entire family by deciding to care for your mental health.

Contrary to what you may have heard, you do not need to breast-feed in order to bond with your baby. If you choose not to breast-feed (for whatever reason), there's no need for concern. You can get even better eye contact with your baby with a bottle in its mouth instead of being squished up face-first into your breast. You can bottle feed bare chested, if you wish, so you and your baby have skin-to-skin contact. You are just as excellent a mother no matter how you choose to feed your baby.

WILL I PASS MY DEPRESSION (OR OTHER MOOD DISORDER) ON TO MY BABY?

Depression and other mood disorders can be passed genetically to offspring just like eye color or any other trait. One of the reasons it's so important for you to be treated to wellness in pregnancy is because, as stated in chapter 6, depression can cross the placenta and affect your developing baby. Often it's difficult to know if a child manifests depression because of a genetic link or because the child has learned depressed behavior from an adult caretaker who's depressed. As long as you're well, you're doing all you can to help your child(ren), and you can feel proud of that. There's nothing more you can do to protect your child from depression if it's genetic, and it's not your fault should it happen. The worst that happens is that you'll make sure your child gets the help he or she needs.

Depression and anxiety disorders are common—many people experience them. In any given year, 25 percent of Americans meet the clinical criteria for a psychiatric disorder, even though most of them don't receive adequate help. Even if you didn't have depression, your child still might. And, of course, even if your child doesn't experience depression, he or she is going to have challenges in life. By caring for yourself, you will have role-modeled empowerment and success in the face of adversity.

Consequences of Untreated Postpartum Depression

It's already been discussed in chapter 6 what can happen if depression in pregnancy isn't treated to complete wellness. Are there also dangers to not treating postpartum depression, or will it go away by itself eventually? Unfortunately, it does not necessarily go away by itself. Untreated postpartum depression can turn into chronic depression. Like any other disorder, the sooner it gets appropriately treated, the sooner you feel better. You deserve to be happy, and your family deserves you to be happy, too. Untreated maternal depression wreaks havoc on marriages and it makes the father more susceptible to depression as well.

Not treating the depression can also affect the child. Infants of depressed moms who are not treated for their postpartum depression are sometimes less active. They may make fewer facial expressions, vocalize less, and tend to be slower to walk. These babies can be fussier, less responsive, and have difficulty interacting. Their heart rates are typically higher, and they often weigh less.

Toddlers who have moms untreated for their depressions have higher risk for mood disorders, poor peer relationships, and have poor self-control. They often exhibit neurological delays and have attention problems. Their behavior starts to look like their mother's depressed behavior.

Preschoolers at three years of age who have had untreated depressed moms are less cooperative and more aggressive. They have less verbal comprehension, lower expressive language skills, and more problem behaviors. They perform poorly on school readiness assessments. One to two months of exposure to severe depression in their moms increases their risk of developing depression by the age of fifteen.

Labor and Delivery Causing Depression, Anxiety, and Trauma

If you've had trauma in your past—emotional, sexual, physical, past childbirth, or other situation—you're at higher risk for experiencing a posttraumatic stress reaction during this upcoming labor and delivery (or postpartum period). The more trauma you've experienced in the past, the higher your risk is. If you're using a birth doula, alert her to this so she'll be tuned in even more sensitively to your needs during labor and delivery. Also, tell your OB so he'll be aware in case you have specific emotional reactions during the process.

Even if trauma is not in your history, make sure to have

someone in the delivery room with you whose job it is to reassure you, communicate with you, and take care of you emotionally. After delivery, make sure you debrief with a nurse, your doctor, or another medical staff member who can answer whatever questions or concerns may be lingering regarding the birth. Sometimes misunderstandings about what methods were used, being upset about treatment, or other perceptions about what happened during labor and delivery can cause unnecessary trauma. If after a couple of weeks there is still emotional upset about the experience—even mild—call a therapist who can help you process what happened, plus give you other suggestions to help your emotional healing.

Prevention of Postpartum Mood Disorders

Although there's no guarantee that you'll be able to avoid a postpartum depression or other postpartum mood or anxiety disorder entirely, there are simple and powerful steps you can take to at least minimize the episode should it occur. All of the elements discussed below should be present in a postpartum plan whether or not you're high risk. All women and couples will benefit from a healthy plan of action. Of course, your plan should be individualized to fit your specific needs, but there are a few basics that need to be in every woman's and couple's plan.

First on the list is the couple discussing wishes and expectations with each other before the baby arrives. "I thought he'd be an involved father" and "My mom made dinner every night, why can't my wife?" are common laments when the couple hasn't communicated before the birth. When each half of the couple assumes how things will be regarding roles, participation, ease of baby care, and so on without communicating these expectations, couples get into trouble. She may be expecting one thing, and he assumes it will be another. When I ask couples if they discussed the sleeping arrangements, for instance, before the baby came, they typically say no. Each is simply assuming that the way he or she is thinking is the way it will be. Bad mistake. It's important not to assume anything, but rather to discuss expectations and desires with your partner.

The other way couples often run into trouble is if the myths surrounding motherhood take over. Realistic expectations are crucial for a happy home. Over the last twenty years of helping new mothers, so many times I've heard things like, "I imagined my life would stay pretty much the same—I'd just take the baby with me," Or, if the mom believes that she shouldn't need any breaks away from her baby, this will lead to burnout, resentment, depression, anxiety, and so on. Making sure to rid yourself of these damaging and totally unrealistic expectations can help you avoid unnecessarily feeling inadequate or like a failure. Other myths include: "when the baby first comes home, it should be the happiest time in my life"; "motherhood is instinctual"; "there's a right way to deliver"; "breast-feeding should be easy," and so forth.

SLEEP

Sleep probably deserves its very own chapter (the way nutrition does), but I'll keep this section short and sweet. Research clearly shows that a solid six-hour chunk of uninterrupted sleep at night will give you an entire sleep cycle (alpha waves, delta waves, REM, and so on). Although six hours is hardly ideal, it will help to prevent sleep deprivation, which can cause mood disorders. Sleep for the new mom in our society is not taken seriously, and that's a problem. Sleep is a medical necessity—not a luxury—*especially* for new moms. Even for those who are not as vulnerable to mood disorders, chronic sleep deprivation can lead to serious health issues. For those who are particularly susceptible to mood problems, sleep needs to be top on the list.

New mothers need to split the nighttime baby care with their partners or another adult support person. If the couple is able, they can hire a night nurse or doula to take over for part of the night. If you're not nursing, a doula, your partner, or another adult can take the whole night a few nights a week, and this will help you in a huge way to prevent postpartum depression and other mood disorders. For more information take a look at *Postpartum Depression for Dummies* (Wiley, 2007) for a simple, practical system that even breast-feeding mothers can use so that sleep at night will be possible. I can't stress enough how important nighttime sleep is for PPD prevention. And just so you know, daytime sleep does not replace nighttime sleep since day sleep doesn't keep your biorhythms normal. That's why people who work swing shifts or night shifts often become depressed. If you're able to nap during the day, set your alarm for thirty minutes (fifteen minutes is ideal). A nap longer than thirty minutes will put you into REM sleep, and this can interfere with your sleep at night.

If you have a damaging myth of motherhood in your head that says, "I'm the mom, so the night responsibility is all up to me," get rid of it fast. It will lead to resentment, exhaustion, depression, burnout, and a host of other issues. Right from the start, set up a schedule of who's going to be on duty when. When you're off duty, sleep in a place where you won't hear the baby at all. And use a fan, air purifier, or other "white noise" to block sound (maybe earplugs, too). Using the "sleep glasses" mentioned in chapter 7 can help you greatly during your shift. When it's your shift, your partner or other adult will wake you up.

NUTRITION

Nutrition is next on the PPD prevention list. Since there is so much to say about the importance of nutrition in managing mood disorders, I devoted a whole chapter (chapter 8) to information about feeding your brain and body the right nutrients to make sure you're feeling the best you can—both physically and emotionally. Refer to that chapter for more information on proper nutrition.

EMOTIONAL SUPPORT

It is imperative that you surround yourself with positive, compassionate, and nonjudgmental people who are willing to support you emotionally, listen to your feelings and concerns, and give you reassurance when you need it at this sensitive time. Some people might want to be included in this close circle, but they don't qualify. If a person has strong opinions as to how you ought to do something (how you should feed the baby, for instance), that's not going to be a good person for you. Look for those individuals who will support your beliefs and wishes so you feel confident—not undermined and belittled. Before your baby pops onto the scene, ask yourself, "who do I have in my life to talk to?" Make a list of those people and put it by your phone, so it will be readily available when you want support.

The healthiest mothers on the planet take good care of themselves in all ways. You need to be first on your list—not last, as many mothers regrettably do (before they burn out). It's your responsibility and duty to keep yourself well, whole, and happy. Your children, marriage, and all other relationships in your life depend on it, so you must make sure it happens. One of the most important pieces of the postpartum wellness plan is to schedule on the calendar regular breaks just for you throughout the week. What works beautifully are four breaks throughout the week for two hours at a time—to nurture yourself (if you're working outside the home, the off-duty times may be fewer, but make them regular). These times are not to be used to do chores or care for the baby. Rather, they are essential chunks of time to remember who you are as a person and to do those activities that nurture you, whatever that means to you. If you love walking your dog, going to lunch with friends, seeing movies, getting a massage, receiving manicures—that's what this time is for. Structure is important, so schedule these breaks on your calendar so they are part of your weekly routine. Whoever will be caring for your baby (and other children) during those times should already be scheduled to come over then. Whether it's your partner, babysitter, relative, or friend—like clockwork, they're on duty, and you're out the door. Refer to *Postpartum Depression for Dummies* (Wiley, 2007) for a more thorough discussion on this topic.

If you're currently working with a therapist, think about increasing the frequency of appointments before delivery and during the first three months postpartum, when the risk for mood disorders presenting is the greatest. If you're taking medication in pregnancy, feeling like you may need it, or exploring your options for medication postpartum just in case, this is the time to see the psychiatrist and make sure you're monitored regularly. Studies (and lots of anecdotal evidence) show that starting medication prior to delivery can prevent another bout of postpartum depression or other mood disorder. If you're high risk and have taken a medication that's worked for you in the past, that would be the one to start taking. If you're using alternative treatment methods either as treatment or prevention, a qualified professional should be monitoring you more frequently as well.

Diagnosis and Treatment: the Usual versus the Ideal

There are no standards as of yet for the diagnosis and treatment of postpartum depression (or the other postpartum mood disorders). Unless you've had a C-section, you don't get checked by the OB until six weeks postpartum, and that visit centers mainly around wound healing, breast-feeding, and birth control. By six weeks, however, many women are already in the midst of a serious postpartum mood disorder. After that, unless there's a problem, you won't see your OB for an entire year.

What would be ideal, and what is beginning to happen in many OB practices, is that every woman is given information about postpartum depression prior to delivery. Screening for depression occurs at least in the third trimester (ideally a quick screening should occur every trimester), and high-risk women are identified before the baby comes and followed up with at two weeks postpartum. All women at the six-week check are screened for postpartum depression and anxiety, and all high-risk women are referred to a therapist to speak with before delivery.

Pediatricians are getting very good at asking the mom (and dad, if he's present) screening questions at the first baby check at two weeks. If the mom shows signs of depression or anxiety, she is referred to a therapist. The pediatrician screens again at the eight-week checkup. Many pediatricians screen parents for mood problems at the well-baby visits at four, six, nine, and twelve months; these are the up-to-date pediatricians who understand that, in order for their patients (kids) to be well, the caretakers of their patients need to be well, too. The great news is that both OBs and pediatricians are definitely moving in the right direction and starting to screen parents, which is making it easier for the entire family to be emotionally healthy.

You now have the tools necessary to ensure your wellness. As you see, there is a wide array of wonderful choices for you. Assemble your support people—both personal and professional—and set up a plan of action that suits your particular physical and emotional needs. Whatever you need to do in order to reach 100 percent, take those steps and feel good about them. Know that you're going to emerge from the pregnancy and postpartum period well, whole, and happy. Here's to your health!

Key Points

- *Even if you are high-risk for postpartum depression, there is much you can do to minimize your risk.*

- *If you are high-risk for postpartum depression, it is wise to have a plan of action ready that can begin immediately postpartum.*

- *With very few exceptions, you can breast-feed your baby even if you are taking a medication.*

RESOURCES

Especially when you're in a vulnerable state of mind and searching for information, it's extra important to be able to rely on solid resources. Instead of surfing the Internet, never knowing what may pop up or whether to trust it, you can instead refer to the following reliable sources.

Using the Internet

When you're anxious, you may be drawn to the Internet, but I don't advise that you use it until you feel more stable. Unless you are visiting specific sites that you know are trustworthy and reliable (like the ones I'm listing here), stay off the Internet. Certain sites and self-professed "experts" can heighten your anxiety. You can always ask a support person to do the searching for you until you feel better.

Web sites

ClearSky-Inc.com, my Web site, provides information on mood disorders in pregnancy as well as resources for new moms and dads. It's geared mainly to the public, but information on training for professionals is listed as well.

Marchofdimes.com/pnhec/188_15663.asp has information on depression in pregnancy on this page.

Pregnancyanddepression.com lists medical articles on all aspects of depression in pregnancy. It's informative, but unless you're used to reading articles in "medical-ese," they can be difficult to wade through.

Womensmentalhealth.org gives you access to up-to-date research on mood disorders, both during pregnancy and postpartum.

4woman.gov/faq/postpartum.htm is sponsored by the U.S. Department of Health and Human Services. The site is reader-friendly and offers information about depression in pregnancy as well as postpartum.

Organizations

Clear Sky Psychology, Inc. (ClearSky-Inc.com). Offers wellness seminars for pregnant and postpartum women. Topics include prevention of mood disorders, various treatments, finding an appropriate therapist, how to tell if you need professional help, communicating your needs to your partner, and more. Professional phone consultations are available, and free literature to download is offered.

Organization of Teratology Specialists (Otispregnancy .org). OTIS is a source of local and national resources and phone numbers that provide information about the safety of medications and other substances for both medical providers and the public.

Postpartum Support International (Postpartum.net). PSI is geared toward social support and offering perinatal resources around the world. PSI's mission is to spread awareness about the emotional changes that women may experience during pregnancy and postpartum. There is an annual conference and a quarterly newsletter for members.

North American Society for Psychosocial Obstetrics and Gynecology (Naspog.org). NASPOG's aim is to encourage scientific clinical research in the field of biopsychosocial factors in obstetric and gynecologic medicine. NASPOG is geared toward researchers and professionals in the field. There is an annual conference, and members receive an annual journal that contains the latest research.

Motherisk (Motherisk.org). This Canadian organization offers a wonderful publication that details the risks and benefits of medications during pregnancy and breast-feeding.

. Further Reading/Viewing

The following three resources are appropriate for both the public and for training professionals.

Bennett, Shoshana S. *Postpartum Depression for Dummies*, Hoboken, New Jersey: Wiley, 2007.

Raffelock, Dean, Robert Rountree, Virginia Hopkins, and Melissa Block. *A Natural Guide to Pregnancy and Postpartum Health.* New York: Avery Publishing, 2002.

Recognizing & Treating Postpartum Depression: A Practitioner's Guide. InjoyVideos.com, 2005.

Support Numbers

Motherisk: (416) 813-6780. This hotline (someone answers) is an excellent resource for pregnant and breast-feeding women. You can ask questions regarding the risk or safety of medications, herbs, diseases, or chemicals.

Postpartum Stressline: (888) 678-2669. All of the trained volunteers on the Stressline are survivors of depression in pregnancy and/or postpartum, and they're looking forward to helping you now that they are recovered. This is a "warm-line," which means you'll leave a message rather than be connected directly to a person, but the volunteer on duty calls you back quickly.

Postpartum Support International: (800) 944-4773. This hotline has a well-trained staff waiting to help you.

GLOSSARY

alpha-linolenic acid (ALA). A type of omega-3 fatty acid found in flax and some vegetable oils.

antidepressant. A medication used to treat depression.

anxiety disorder. A condition that produces excessive worry and fear about everyday situations.

benzodiazipines. A class of drugs used to treat anxiety.

bipolar disorder. A mood disorder, also known as manic-depressive illness, that causes extreme shifts from severe depression to abnormally elevated mood.

clinical experience. Expertise gained from actually working hands-on, as opposed to learning only from books.

contraindication. A situation where the use of a particular treatment is not advisable.

docosahexanoic acid (DHA). An essential fatty acid necessary for brain health and infant development.

dopamine. A neurotransmitter (brain chemical).

doula. A woman trained to help a woman/couple through labor, delivery, and postpartum.

eicosapentenoic acid (EPA). An essential fatty acid important for brain and nerve function.

estrogen. A group of hormones functioning as the primary female sex hormone.

glycemic index. A ranking of carbohydrate foods based on the effect each has on blood sugar.

homeopathy. An alternative medical system that treats the symptoms of a disease with tiny doses of a natural substance.

MAOIs, *see* monoamine oxidase inhibitors.

midwife. A person trained to assist a woman during childbirth.

monoamine oxidase inhibitors. A class of antidepressant drugs that are not frequently used.

mood disorder. A type of illness characterized by severe or prolonged mood states that disrupt the person's daily functioning.

mood stabilizer. A psychiatric medication used to treat mood disorders, especially bipolar disorder.

neural tube defect. A congenital defect of the brain and spinal cord.

obsessive compulsive disorder. An anxiety disorder that causes recurrent, unwanted thoughts (obsessions) or rituals (compulsions) that those suffering feel they cannot control.

OCD, *see* obsessive compulsive disorder.

omega-3 fatty acids. Essential fatty acids necessary to human health, but they cannot be manufactured by the body.

perinatal mood disorder. A mood disorder occurring during the time period that includes pregnancy and up to one year after delivery.

PMDD, *see* premenstrual dysphoric disorder.

postpartum depression A serious medical condition that occurs in the months following delivery.

postpartum psychosis. A mental illness that involves the rapid onset of psychotic symptoms in a woman following childbirth.

PPD, *see* postpartum depression.

premenstrual dysphoric disorder. A disorder that severely affects emotions and the ability to function; it surfaces between ovulation and menstruation.

PPP, *see* postpartum psychosis.

progesterone. A very important hormone produced in the female body that helps to regulate the menstrual cycle.

psychosis. A mental state involving being out of touch with reality.

psychotherapy. The treatment of emotional or behavioral problems by psychological means.

psychotropic drug. Any drug capable of affecting the mind, behavior, or emotions.

selective serotonin reuptake inhibitors. A newer class of antidepressant drugs.

serotonin. A neurotransmitter (brain chemical) that helps regulate sleep, appetite, moods, and pain.

SSRIs, *see* selective serotonin reuptake inhibitors.

TCAs, *see* tricyclic antidepressants.

tricyclic antidepressants. An older class of antidepressant drugs.

METRIC CONVERSION TABLES

APPROXIMATE U.S.–METRIC EQUIVALENTS

LIQUID INGREDIENTS

U.S. MEASURES	METRIC	U.S. MEASURES	METRIC
¼ tsp.	1.23 ml	2 Tbsp.	29.57 ml
½ tsp.	2.36 ml	3 Tbsp.	44.36 ml
¾ tsp.	3.70 ml	¼ cup	59.15 ml
1 tsp.	4.93 ml	½ cup	118.30 ml
1¼ tsp.	6.16 ml	1 cup	236.59 ml
1½ tsp.	7.39 ml	2 cups or 1 pt.	473.18 ml
1¾ tsp.	8.63 ml	3 cups	709.77 ml
2 tsp.	9.86 ml	4 cups or 1 qt.	946.36 ml
1 Tbsp.	14.79 ml	4 qts. or 1 gal.	3.79 lt

DRY INGREDIENTS

U.S. MEASURES	METRIC		U.S. MEASURES	METRIC
17³⁄₅ oz.	1 livre	500 g	2 oz.	60 (56.6) g
16 oz.	1 lb.	454 g	1¾ oz.	50 g
8⅞ oz.		250 g	1 oz.	30 (28.3) g
5¼ oz.		150 g	⅞ oz.	25 g
4½ oz.		125 g	¾ oz.	21 (21.3) g
4 oz.		115 (113.2) g	½ oz.	15 (14.2) g
3½ oz.		100 g	¼ oz.	7 (7.1) g
3 oz.		85 (84.9) g	⅛ oz.	3½ (3.5) g
2⅘ oz.		80 g	¹⁄₁₆ oz.	2 (1.8) g

INDEX

MAOIs (monoamine oxidase inhibitors), 132
massage therapists (L.M.T.s), 158–59
media, 144–46
medications
  antianxiety, 132–37
  antidepressants, 128–32
  antipsychotics, 141
  baby's exposure to, 42–43
  birth defects and, 13–14
  breast-feeding and, 150–51, 217–18
  commonality of prescriptions for, 117, 118–19
  dangers of discontinuing, 40–43
  doctors and pharmaceutical industry, 119–20
  dosages, 132, 143
  drug classifications, 122–25
  drug development, 123–24
  FDA classifications, 122, 124–25
  guilt and, 26
  health testing and, 135–36
  importance of continuing, 5–6, 31, 39
  Lynda's story, 6–12
  media and, 144–46
  medical data, 77–78

mood stabilizers, 139–42
  over-the-counter, 149–50
  as part of solution, 50, 51
  as part of treatment plan, 120–21
  purposes of, 117–18
  relapse and, 39–40
  research methods, 127–28
  risks of not taking, 116–17
  risks *vs.* benefits, 25–26
  self-care and, 117
  sleep aids, 137–39
  stigma about taking, 94–95
  switching, 28–29, 147–49
  testing on pregnant women, 143
  when partner is against, 79–82
  See also alternative treatments; antidepressants; decision-making; drugs
melatonin, 159, 178–79
metric conversion tables, 236
midwives, 54
monoamine oxidase inhibitors (MAOIs), 132
mood disorders
  appetite and, 99
  bipolar disorder, 139, 146, 150–51

ABOUT THE AUTHOR

Shoshana Bennett, Ph.D., is the author of *Postpartum Depression for Dummies* and co-author of *Beyond the Blues: Understanding and Treating Prenatal and Postpartum Depression*. She's also created guided imagery audios that are specifically focused on helping moms take care of themselves. She is a consultant for numerous news stations and the postpartum expert for ABC's *20/20* and other national TV shows. She's interviewed regularly on radio and hosts her own show "Mom's Health Matters." Feature articles on her work have been published in the *San Francisco Chronicle* and the *San Jose Mercury News* and she has been quoted in hundreds of newspapers and magazines such as the *Boston Globe, Glamour, Psychology Today, New York Post, Self, Cosmopolitan, Women's Day, Parents Magazine, USA Weekend*, and the *Chicago Tribune*.

Dr. Shoshana is a survivor of two life-threatening, undiagnosed postpartum depressions. A highly regarded pioneer in the field, she founded Postpartum Assistance for Mothers in 1987, and is a former president of Postpartum Support International. Dr. Shoshana has helped over 17,000 women worldwide through individual consultations, support groups, and wellness seminars. A noted guest lecturer and keynote speaker, she travels throughout the United States and abroad, training medical and mental health professionals to assess and treat postpartum depression and related mood disorders. She earned three teaching credentials, two master's degrees, and a Ph.D., and is a licensed clinical psychologist. She is working to pass legislation that helps reduce the incidence and impact of perinatal mood disorders. She can be contacted for consultations and speaking engagements through ClearSky-Inc .com.